The Cancer Recovery Healthy Exchanges® Cookbook

A HEALTHY EXCHANGES® COOKBOOK

JoAnna M. Lund
with Barbara Alpert

Introduction by
Catherine Muha, R.N., M.S.N.

HELPing Others HELP Themselves
the **Healthy Exchanges**® Way™

A Perigee Book

A Perigee Book
Published by The Berkley Publishing Group
A division of Penguin Putnam Inc.
375 Hudson Street
New York, New York 10014

For more information about Healthy Exchanges products, contact:
Healthy Exchanges, Inc.
P.O. Box 124
DeWitt, Iowa 52742-0124
(319) 659-8234

First edition: March 2000

Published simultaneously in Canada.

The Penguin Putnam Inc. World Wide Web site address is
http://www.penguinputnam.com

Library of Congress Cataloging-in-Publication Data

Lund, JoAnna M.
    The cancer recovery healthy exchanges cookbook / JoAnna M. Lund with Barbara
Alpert ; introduction by Catherine Muha.—1st ed.
        p. cm
    "A healthy exchanges cookbook."
    "A Perigee book."
    Includes index.
    ISBN 0-399-52576-9
    1. Cancer—Diet therapy—Recipes.   2. Food exchange lists.   I. Alpert, Barbara.
II. Title.

RC271.D52 L86 2000
641.5'631—dc21
                                                                99-055709
                                                                CIP

Printed in the United States of America

10   9   8   7   6   5   4   3   2   1

This cookbook is dedicated in loving memory to my parents, Jerome and Agnes McAndrews, who taught me to persevere even through rough times. It is also dedicated to everyone whose life has been touched in any way by cancer. Maybe you are a survivor yourself, or maybe you are a caregiver for someone who is currently going through treatment, or maybe you are a neighborly shoulder to lean on when a friend first learns that she has cancer.

In any case, you quickly learn that *food just doesn't taste like it used to*. I hope that by sharing my "common folk" healthy recipes, you and your loved ones can again experience the simple enjoyment of eating everyday meals. An elderly Texas gentleman who was recovering from cancer proclaimed my recipes to be "dang good groceries." I don't think I could have described them better myself!

My mother, who was as prolific with poetry as I am with recipes, wrote this beautiful poem several years ago. Her words are as timely today as they were the day she composed them. May this poem be of comfort to you and your loved ones in your time of need.

In His Care

Everything seemed to be in turmoil,
    I was consumed with despair.
Like a storm, dark clouds gathered around me,
    shutting out light everywhere.
Nothing seemed to bring me help or comfort,
    the worry was too much to bear,
Until I knelt at the foot of His cross
    and asked Him for help through prayer.

—Agnes Carrington McAndrews

Contents

Acknowledgments

When I changed my prayer from what I wanted to what I needed, my prayers were answered in ways I never could have imagined. God gives us all talents to use for the betterment of others. Mine happens to be creating "common folk" healthy recipes and sharing a commonsense approach to healthy living. For helping me share my talents with others, I want to thank:

Doctors and dietitians all over America, for suggesting my cookbooks to their patients, because they know my recipes are low enough in fats, sugars, and sodium to be healthy, but *just* high enough to be tasty.

Catherine Muha, R.N., M.S.N., for sharing her commonsense suggestions and advice for coping with cancer.

Rose Hoenig, R.D., L.D., for answering my nutritional questions in words I can understand, and for calculating the Diabetic Exchanges.

John Duff, not only for editing my current books but for encouraging me to create continually both new recipes and new ideas.

Angela Miller and Coleen O'Shea, for being the kind of agents that other authors only dream about finding someday.

Barbara Alpert, for taking my recipes, my words, and my concepts, and making them even better as we turn them into manuscripts.

Shirley Morrow, Lori Hansen, Rita Ahlers, and Cheryl Sommers, for assisting me in getting my recipes "just right" as they help type, calculate, and test them (and yes, sometimes even do my dishes!).

Cliff Lund, for grabbing onto my dream of sharing my recipes with all his might and helping me with just about everything except those dishes.

God, for bestowing on me in my time of need the ability to create "common folk" healthy recipes and to write in a "Grandma Moses" style, then showing me how to help others with those talents as I help myself.

Introduction

by Catherine A. Muha, R.N., M.S.N.

Your diet is an important part of your treatment for cancer. Eating the right kinds of foods before, during, and after your treatment can help you feel better and stay stronger. Your doctor, nurse, or a registered dietitian can explain in more detail why eating well is so vital to the success of your treatment, and a healthy cookbook like this one can help you meet those nutritional needs.

It's equally important to get your information from reliable sources. The advice I've gathered in this section reflects the tried-and-true experiences of many cancer patients and the doctors, nurses, and dietitians who work with them.

Let me begin with a definition. Cancer is a group of more than one hundred different diseases. It occurs when cells become abnormal and keep dividing and forming new cells without control or order. If cells keep dividing when new cells are not needed, a mass of tissue forms. This mass of extra tissue, called a growth or tumor, can be benign (not cancer) or malignant (cancer).

Generally, the sooner your cancer is diagnosed and treated, the better your chances for a full recovery. Talk with your doctor about your cancer risk and what problems to watch for, and stick to a schedule of regular checkups. Your doctor's advice will consider your age, medical history, and other risk factors. If you have specific concerns, don't delay getting a doctor's opinion—early diagnosis is key.

Before Treatment Begins

When your cancer was first diagnosed, your doctor talked to you about a treatment plan. This may have involved surgery, radiation therapy, chemotherapy, hormone therapy, and biologic therapy (immunotherapy), or some combination of those treatments. All these methods of treating cancer kill cells. In the process of killing the cancer cells, some healthy cells are also damaged. That is what causes the side effects of cancer treatment. Side effects that can affect your ability to eat include loss of appetite, changes in weight (either losing or gaining weight), sore mouth or throat, dry mouth, dental and gum problems, changes in sense of taste or smell, nausea, vomiting, diarrhea, lactose intolerance, constipation, and fatigue or depression.

You may or may not experience any of these side effects. Many factors determine whether you will have any and how severe they will be. These factors include your overall health, the type of cancer you have, the part of your body being treated, the type and length of treatment, and the dose of treatment. The good news is that if you do have side effects, they can often be controlled. Most side effects go away after treatment ends. Also, there are new drugs designed to control such side effects, and they work well. Before treatment begins, ask questions about what to expect; you'll feel better able to handle what follows.

Preparing Yourself for Cancer Treatment

Until your treatment actually starts, it's hard to know exactly what, if any, side effects you may have or how you'll feel. Why not begin by thinking of your treatment as a time for you to concentrate on yourself and on getting well? Here are some other ways to get ready:

Think Positively

- Starting with a positive attitude, talking out your feelings, becoming well-informed about your cancer and treatment, and planning ways to cope can all help reduce worry and anxiety, make you feel more in control, and help you keep your appetite.

- Try to spend more time with people who make you feel good about yourself.

- Ask for help when you need it. Everyone needs support sometimes; facing your situation alone can be tiring and frightening.

Eat a Healthy Diet and Live a Healthy Lifestyle

- A healthy diet is vital for your body to work at its best. This is even more important when you're being treated for cancer. If you've been eating a healthy diet, you'll go into treatment with reserves to help keep up your strength, prevent body tissue from breaking down, rebuild tissue, and maintain your defenses against infection.

- People who eat well are better able to cope with side effects. You may even be able to handle higher doses of certain treatments. We know that some cancer treatments are actually more effective if patients are well-nourished and getting enough calories and protein in their diets.

- Be open-minded about trying new foods. Some things you may never have liked before may taste good to you during your treatment. This cookbook is filled with a variety of tasty new dishes to choose from.

- Don't smoke or chew tobacco.

- Consider changes to your lifestyle that will help you cope better. Sufficient sleep is especially important!

Plan Ahead

- Stock the pantry and freezer with your favorite foods so that you won't need to shop as often. Include foods you know you can eat even when you feel sick.

- Keep foods handy that need little or no preparation: pudding, peanut butter, tuna fish, cheese, and eggs, for example.

- Do some cooking in advance and freeze in meal-sized portions. Many of JoAnna's recipes can be prepared in advance, with extra servings frozen for easy reheating.

- Ask family or friends for help with shopping or cooking. Or, ask them to manage that job for you.

- Talk to a registered dietitian about your concerns, and ask for ideas and help in planning meals. Develop a grocery list together that includes foods that might help with potential side effects, such as constipation or nausea. Find out what has worked for other patients.

Managing Eating Problems During Treatment

All the methods of treating cancer—surgery, radiation therapy, chemotherapy, hormone therapy, and biological therapy (immunotherapy)—are very powerful. Although these treatments target the fastest-growing cancer cells in your body, healthy cells can also be damaged. Healthy cells that normally grow and divide rapidly, such as those of the mouth, digestive tract, and hair, are often affected by cancer treatments. This damage to healthy cells can produce unpleasant side effects and cause eating problems.

The part of the body being treated, the type and length of treatment, and the dose of treatment determine whether side effects will occur and what they might be.

Some eating problems are caused by the treatment itself. Other times, patients may have trouble eating because they are upset, worried, or afraid. Losing your appetite and nausea are two normal responses to feeling nervous or fearful. Once you get into your treatment period, you'll have a better sense of what may happen and how you will react, and any anxiety-related eating problems should improve.

While you are in the hospital or undergoing treatment, your doctors, nurses, or dietitian can answer your questions and give you suggestions for specific meals, snacks, and food choices. If you're experiencing eating problems, make sure they know about it. They can also help you handle dietary preferences unique to your cultural and ethnic background. Continue to call on them for guidance if problems arise during your recovery.

Recommendations about food and eating for cancer patients can be very different from the usual suggestions for healthful eating. This can be confusing for many patients, because such suggestions may seem to be the opposite of what they've always heard. Most nutrition guidelines stress eating lots of fruits, vegetables, and whole-grain breads and cereals; they also suggest including moderate amounts of meat and dairy products and cutting back on fat, sugar, alcohol, and salt.

But recommendations for cancer patients may ask you to eat higher-calorie foods that are high in protein. These may include eating or drinking more milk, or adding cream, cheese, and cooked eggs to the menu. They may suggest using more sauces and gravies, or changing your cooking methods to include more butter, margarine, or oil. Sometimes, nutrition recommendations for cancer patients suggest that you cut back on certain high-fiber foods because these foods can aggravate problems such as diarrhea or a sore mouth.

Why are nutrition recommendations for cancer patients different? Because they are designed to build up your strength and help you withstand the effects of your cancer and its treatment. When you are healthy, eating enough food to get the nutrients you need is usually not a problem. During cancer treatment, however, this can become a challenge, especially if you're experiencing side effects or simply don't feel well.

It's important to remember that there aren't any hard and fast nutrition rules during cancer treatment. Some patients may continue to enjoy eating and experience a normal appetite throughout treatment. Others may have days when they don't feel like eating at all, days when even the thought of food may make them feel ill. Here are some things to keep in mind:

- When you can eat, try to eat meals and snacks with sufficient protein and calories. This will help you keep up your strength, prevent body tissues from breaking down, and rebuild tissues that cancer treatment may harm.

- Many patients find that their appetite is better in the morning. If this is true for you, take advantage of it and eat more then.

- Try new recipes—like the ones in this cookbook!

- If you don't feel well and can eat only one or two things, stick with them until you are able to eat other foods. Try a liquid meal replacement for extra calories and protein. If you don't like the taste of one brand, keep trying to find one that appeals to you.

- On those days when you can't eat at all, don't worry about it. Do what you can to make yourself feel better. Come back to eating as soon as you can, and let your doctor know if this problem doesn't get better within a couple of days.

- Try to drink plenty of fluids, especially on those days when you don't feel like eating. Water is essential to your body's proper functioning, so getting enough fluids will ensure that your body has the water it needs. For most adults, 6 to 8 cups of fluid a day is a good target. Try carrying a water bottle with you during the day.

Coping with Side Effects

Loss of Appetite

Loss of appetite or poor appetite is one of the most common problems that occurs with cancer and its treatment. No one knows exactly what causes loss of appetite. It may be caused by the treatments or by the cancer itself. Emotions such as fear or depression can also take away your appetite. Sometimes the side effects of treatment, such as nausea, vomiting, or changes in food's taste or smell, make you feel like not eating. Often, loss of appetite happens for just a day or two; for some, it's an ongoing concern. Whatever the reason, here are some suggestions that may help:

- Try liquid or powdered meal replacements, such as "instant breakfast" mix, during times when it is hard for you to eat regular food.

- Try eating frequent small meals throughout the day, rather than three big ones. It may be easier to eat more that way, and you won't get so full.

- Keep snacks within easy reach so you can have something whenever you feel like it. Cheese and crackers, muffins, ice cream, peanut butter, fruit, and pudding are good possibilities.

- Even if you don't feel like eating solid foods, try to drink beverages during the day. Juice, soup, and other fluid foods can provide important calories and nutrients.

- Sometimes, changing the form of a food will make it more appetizing and help you eat better. For example, if eating whole fresh fruit is a problem, try mixing fruit into a milkshake.

- Try eating softer, cool, or frozen foods, such as yogurt, milkshakes, or popsicles.

- During meals, sip only small amounts of liquid, because drinking may fill you up before you've had a chance to eat very much.

- Make mealtimes as relaxed as possible. Presenting food or meals in an attractive way may also help.

- If your doctor allows, have a small glass of wine or beer during a meal. It may help to stimulate your appetite.

- Regular exercise may help your appetite. Check with your doctor to see what options are open to you.

Weight Loss

Many cancer patients lose weight during their cancer treatment. This is partly due to the effects of the cancer on the body. But you may also lose weight if you have little appetite and are eating less than usual because of your treatment or emotional worries. Whatever the reason, talk with your doctor, nurse, or dietitian about how to increase calories and protein in your diet, and review the suggestions at the end of this section.

Weight Gain

Some patients find their weight does not change during treatment. They may even gain weight. This is particularly true for breast, prostate, and ovarian cancer patients taking certain medications or who are on hormone therapy or chemotherapy.

It is important *not* to go on a diet right away if you notice weight gain. Instead, tell your doctor so you can find out what may be causing this change. Sometimes, weight gain happens because certain anti-cancer drugs cause your body to hold on to excess fluid. This condition is called edema. The weight comes from the extra water. If this is the case, your doctor may suggest you talk to a registered dietitian about how to limit the amount of salt you eat. This is important because salt causes your body to hold extra water.

Weight gain may also occur as the result of increased appetite and eating more calories than your body can use. If this is the case, and you want to stop gaining weight, here are some tips that can help.

- Emphasize fruits, vegetables, and breads and cereals.

- Choose lean meats (lean beef or pork trimmed of fat, chicken without skin) and low-fat dairy products (skim or 1% milk, light yogurt).

- Cut back on added butter, mayonnaise, sweets (except for JoAnna's desserts!), and other extras.

- Choose low-fat and low-calorie cooking methods (broiling, steaming).

- If you feel up to it, increase the amount of exercise you do.

Sore Mouth or Throat

Mouth sores, tender gums, and a sore throat or esophagus often result from radiation therapy, chemotherapy, or infection. If you have a sore mouth or gums, see your doctor to be sure the soreness is a treatment side effect and not an unrelated dental problem. The doctor may be able to give you medicine that will control mouth and throat pain. Your dentist also can give you tips on caring for your mouth.

Certain foods will irritate an already tender mouth and make chewing and swallowing difficult. By carefully choosing the foods you eat and by taking good care of your mouth, teeth, and gums, you can usually make eating easier. Here are some suggestions:

- Try soft foods that are easy to chew and swallow, such as milkshakes, bananas and other fruit, macaroni and cheese, puddings, scrambled eggs, and pureed foods.

- Avoid foods or liquids that can irritate your mouth. These include oranges or other citrus fruit/juices; tomato sauces; spicy or salty foods; raw vegetables; coarse foods like crackers; and commercial mouthwashes that contain alcohol.

- Cook foods until they are soft and tender, and then cut them into small pieces.

- Use a blender or food processor to puree food.

- Mix food with butter or sauce to make it easier to swallow.

- Try eating foods cold or at room temperature. Hot foods can irritate a tender mouth.

- Try sucking on ice chips.

- If your teeth and gums are sore, your dentist may be able to recommend a special product for cleaning your teeth.

- Rinse your mouth often with water to remove food and bacteria and to promote healing.

- Ask your doctor about anesthetic lozenges and sprays that can numb your mouth and throat long enough for you to eat meals.

Dry Mouth

Chemotherapy and radiation therapy in the head or neck area can reduce the flow of saliva and cause dry mouth. When this happens, foods are harder to chew and swallow. Also, dry mouth can change the way foods taste. Some of the ideas listed under "Sore Mouth or Throat" may help, as well as these suggestions:

- Have a sip of water every few minutes to help you swallow and talk more easily. Carry a water bottle with you.

- Suck on hard candy or a popsicle, or chew gum. These can help produce more saliva.

- Keep your lips moist with lip salves.

- If your dry mouth problem is severe, ask your doctor or dentist about products that coat, protect, and moisten your mouth and throat. These are sometimes called "artificial saliva."

Dental and Gum Problems

Cancer and cancer treatment can cause tooth decay and other problems for your teeth and gums. For example, radiation to the mouth can affect your salivary glands, making your mouth dry and increasing your risk of cavities. Your doctor and dentist should work closely together to fix any problems with your teeth before you start treatment. Brushing after each meal or snack is a good idea. Here are some other ideas for preventing dental problems:

- Be sure to see your dentist regularly. Cancer patients may need to be seen more often than usual.

- Use a soft toothbrush.

- Rinse your mouth with warm water when your gums and mouth are sore.

Changed Sense of Taste or Smell

Your sense of smell or taste may change during your illness or treatment. Some foods, especially meat or other high-protein choices, may begin to have a bitter or metallic taste. Many foods will have less taste. For most people, these changes in taste and smell go away when their treatment is finished. There is no foolproof way to prevent changes to your sense of taste or smell because each person is affected differently by illness and treatments. However, these tips should help:

- Choose and prepare foods that look and smell good to you.

- "Help" the flavor of the meat, chicken, or fish by marinating it in sweet fruit juices, Italian dressing, or other tasty mixtures.

- Try using small amounts of flavorful seasonings, such as basil, oregano, or rosemary.

- If smells bother you, try serving foods at room temperature, turning on the kitchen fan, covering foods when cooking, and cooking outdoors when possible.

- Try using bacon, ham, or onion to add flavor to vegetables.

Nausea

Nausea, with or without vomiting, is a common side effect of cancer treatment. Some people experience nausea and vomiting right after treatment; others don't have it until two or three days later. Many people never experience nausea, and for those who do, nausea often goes away once treatment is completed. Also, there are now drugs that can effectively control this side effect. These medications, called anti-emetics, are often given at the beginning of a chemotherapy session to prevent nausea. If nausea is a concern for you, try these tips:

- Ask your doctor about medications that might help you control nausea and vomiting.

- Choose foods that are easy on the stomach: toast, crackers, yogurt, sherbet, angel food cake, cream of wheat or oatmeal, boiled potatoes, noodles, rice, canned fruit, clear liquids, ice chips, or carbonated drinks.

- Avoid foods that are fatty, greasy, or fried; are sweet, like candy, cookies, or cake; are spicy or hot; or have strong odors.

- Eat small amounts, often and slowly.

- Avoid eating in a room that's stuffy or warm, or one that has odors that might disagree with you.

- Drink fewer liquids with meals.

- Have foods and drinks at room temperature or cooler, as hot foods may add to the nausea.

- Don't force yourself to eat when you feel nauseated.

- Rest after meals, because activity may slow digestion. It's best to rest sitting up for about an hour after meals.

- If nausea is a problem in the morning, try eating dry toast or crackers before getting up.

- Wear loose-fitting clothes.

- Try to keep track of when your nausea occurs and what causes it (specific foods, events, surroundings). Change your diet and schedule as needed.

Vomiting
Vomiting may follow nausea and may be brought on by a particular treatment, food odors, gas in the stomach or bowel, or motion. In some people, certain associations or surroundings (such as the hospital) may cause vomiting. As with nausea, some people have vomiting right after treatment, while others don't have it until a day

or more later. Again, talk with your doctor about medications that will help control vomiting.

Very often, if you control nausea, you can prevent vomiting. At times, though, you may not be able to prevent either. Relaxation exercises or meditation may help you. These usually involve deep rhythmic breathing and quiet concentration, and can be done almost anywhere. If vomiting does occur, try these suggestions to help prevent further episodes:

- Do not eat or drink anything until you have the vomiting under control.

- Once the vomiting is under control, try small amounts of clear liquids, such as water or bouillon.

- When you are able to keep down clear liquids, try a full-liquid diet or a soft diet. Continue taking small amounts as often as you can keep them down. If you feel okay, gradually work up to your regular diet.

Diarrhea

Diarrhea may have several causes, including chemotherapy, radiation therapy to the abdomen, infection, food sensitivities, and emotional upset. Work with your doctor to identify the cause of your diarrhea so that it can be successfully treated.

During diarrhea, food passes quickly through the bowel before your body has a chance to absorb enough vitamins, minerals, and water. This may cause problems such as dehydration, which means that your body does not have enough water to work well. Long-term or severe diarrhea is especially problematic, so contact your doctor if the diarrhea is severe or lasts for more than a couple of days. Here are some ideas for coping with diarrhea:

- Drink plenty of fluids to replenish what you lose with the diarrhea.

- Eat small amounts of food throughout the day instead of three large meals.

- Eat plenty of foods and liquids that contain sodium and potassium, two important minerals that help your body work properly. These minerals are often lost during diarrhea.

Good high-sodium liquids include bouillon or fat-free broth. Foods high in potassium that don't cause diarrhea include bananas, peach and apricot nectar, and boiled or mashed potatoes. Sports drinks contain both sodium and potassium and have easily absorbable forms of carbohydrates.

- Try these foods: yogurt, rice, noodles, pasta, cream of wheat, smooth peanut butter, white bread, well-cooked vegetables, canned or peeled fruits, skinned chicken or turkey, lean beef, and fish.

- Avoid greasy, fatty, or fried foods; raw vegetables and their skins; and high-fiber vegetables such as broccoli, corn, dried beans, cabbage, peas, and cauliflower.

- Limit foods and drinks that contain caffeine, such as coffee, some sodas, and chocolate.

- Avoid very hot or cold foods and beverages. Drink liquids that are at room temperature.

Lactose Intolerance

Lactose intolerance means that your body can't digest or absorb the milk sugar called lactose. Milk, other milk-based dairy products (such as cheese and ice cream), and foods to which milk has been added (such as pudding) may contain lactose.

Lactose intolerance may occur after some cancer treatments. If you have this problem, your doctor may advise you to follow a diet that is low in foods that contain lactose. Talk to a registered dietitian to get advice and specific tips about how to follow a low-lactose diet. Your supermarket should carry milk and other products that have been modified to reduce or eliminate the lactose.

Constipation

Some anti-cancer drugs and other drugs, such as pain medications, may cause constipation. This problem also can occur if your diet lacks enough fluid or fiber, or if you've been in bed for a long time. Here are some suggestions for preventing and treating constipation:

- Drink plenty of fluids—at least eight 8-ounce glasses every day. This will help to keep your stools soft.

- Have a hot drink about one-half hour before your usual time for a bowel movement.

- Check with your doctor to see if you can increase the fiber in your diet.

- Get some exercise every day. Find out about the amount and type of exercise that's right for you.

- If needed, ask your doctor about medications to help ease constipation. Be sure to check with your doctor before taking any laxatives or stool softeners.

Fatigue and Depression

All the methods of treating cancer are powerful, and these treatments may go on for weeks, months, or even years. They may even cause more illness and discomfort than the initial disease. Many patients say they feel exhausted, depressed, or unable to concentrate. Fatigue during cancer treatment can be related to a number of causes: not eating, inactivity, low blood counts, depression, poor sleep, and side effects of medicine. It is important for you to raise the issue with your health-care team if you are experiencing fatigue. Together, you can determine what is causing the problem and make adjustments, since many of the causes can be treated.

Fatigue and depression aren't eating problems as such, but they can affect your interest in food and compromise your ability to shop and prepare healthy meals. Here are some suggestions that may help:

- Talk about your feelings and your fears. Being open about your emotions can make them seem more manageable. Share your thoughts with your nurse or social worker, who can help you find ways to lessen your worries and cope with your fears.

- Become familiar with your treatment, possible side effects, and ways of coping. Becoming knowledgeable and acting on that knowledge will help you feel more in control.

- Make sure you get enough rest. Take several naps or rest breaks during the day; try easier or shorter versions of your usual activities.

- Take short walks or get regular exercise, if possible. Some people find this helps to lessen their fatigue and raise their spirits.

Keeping Track of Side Effects

It's important to keep track of eating-related side effects you experience while you're undergoing cancer treatment. Develop your own weekly tracking form to use for writing down this information:

Name:
Week of:
Type and date of your last treatment(s):
Your weight: (measure once a week)
List of eating-related side effects that you may experience: (dry mouth, nausea, fatigue, etc.) Next to each side effect, note the day and severity of the side effect (1=mild, 2=moderate, 3=severe)
Other questions and concerns: (keep a list of questions you want to ask your doctor)

It may be helpful to keep the tracking forms in a notebook that you can bring with you each time you see your doctor.

Special Notes for Caregivers

There is much that you can do to help your friend or loved one through the period of cancer treatment. Review the tips in the previous sections; they can provide some useful insights when you prepare meals and snacks for the patient. Here are some other ideas to help you cope:

- Be prepared for the patient's tastes to change from day to day. Some days he or she will refuse favorite foods because they just don't taste good. Other times, a dish that couldn't be tolerated just the day before is suddenly appealing.

- Have food within easy reach at home (like snacks at the bedside).

- Prepare food in advance so it is easy to heat up and serve when the patient is ready.

- Be prepared for times when the patient is able to eat only one or two foods for a few days in a row, until side effects diminish. Even if he or she can't eat, still encourage plenty of fluids.

- Talk about needs and concerns, and get the patient's ideas about what might work best. This willingness in a caregiver to be flexible and supportive, no matter what, will help the patient feel more in control of the situation.

- Encourage and support without being overwhelming.

After Cancer Treatment Ends

Most eating-related side effects associated with cancer treatment go away after treatment ends. If you have experienced side effects, you should gradually begin to feel better, and your interest in food and mealtimes will return. Sometimes, though, side effects persist, especially weight loss. If this happens to you, talk with your doctor and work out a plan together to address the problem.

After cancer treatment ends and you're feeling better, you may want to think again about the traditional guidelines for healthy eating. Just as you wanted to go into treatment with all the reserves that such a diet could give you, you'll want to do the best you can at this important time. There's no current research to confirm that the foods you eat will *prevent* your cancer from recurring. But we do know that eating right will help you regain your strength, rebuild tissue, and feel well. Here are some basics:

- Focus on eating a variety of food every day. No one food contains all the nutrients you require.

- Emphasize fruits and vegetables. Raw or cooked vegetables, fruits, and fruit juices provide the vitamins, minerals, and fiber you need.

- Emphasize breads and cereals, especially the whole-grain variety, such as whole-wheat bread, oats, and brown rice.

These foods are good sources of complex carbohydrates, vitamins and minerals, and fiber.

- Go easy on fat, salt, sugar, alcohol, and smoked or pickled foods. Choose low-fat milk products, and consume small portions (no more than 6 to 7 ounces a day) of lean meat and poultry without skin. Try lower-fat cooking methods, such as broiling, steaming and poaching.

- Don't eat charred foods.

- Don't smoke or chew tobacco.

Some patients need to have treatments that last a long time. Others may have surgery to remove part of the stomach or intestines. These patients may experience ongoing eating-related concerns. If this is true for you, your doctor and a registered dietitian can discuss the long-term issues you will be facing. Together, you can develop an individual diet plan that satisfies your needs.

Getting Back into Eating
Even once your treatment is over and you're feeling much better, you still may not feel "back to your old self." Here are some ways to help you ease back into regular meals and mealtimes:

- Make simple meals using familiar, easy-to-prepare recipes.

- Cook enough for two or three meals, then freeze the remainder for later.

- Take advantage of the supermarket's salad bar and prepared foods to make cooking easier.

- Think again about ways you used to make mealtime special—music, attractive table settings—and try them again.

- Be willing to ask a friend or family member for help with cooking or shopping.

Special Issues

Commercial Products to Improve Nutrition

If you cannot get enough calories and protein from your diet, commercial meal replacements such as drinks, shakes, and "instant breakfast" powders may help. Other products also can be added to any food or beverage. These supplements are high in protein and calories and have extra vitamins and minerals. They come in liquid, pudding, and powder forms. Most of these products need no refrigeration until you open them. That means you can carry them with you and have them whenever you feel hungry or thirsty. They are also good chilled as between-meal or bedtime snacks. Many supermarkets and drugstores carry a variety of commercial liquid meal replacements.

Preventing Food-Borne Illness

Cancer patients undergoing treatment can develop a weakened immune system, because most anti-cancer drugs decrease the body's ability to make white blood cells, the cells that fight infection. That's why cancer patients should be especially careful to avoid infections and food-borne illnesses. Here are some tips to help you prevent food-borne illness:

- Wash all raw fruits and vegetables well. If something can't be well washed (like raspberries), avoid it. Scrub rough surfaces, like the skin of a melon, prior to cutting.

- Carefully wash your hands and food preparation surfaces (knives, cutting boards) before and after preparing food, especially after handling raw meat.

- Refrigerate perishable foods as soon as possible.

- Thaw meat in the refrigerator, not on the kitchen counter.

- Be sure to cook meat and eggs thoroughly.

- Avoid raw shellfish and use only pasteurized or processed ciders and juices and pasteurized milk and cheese.

Will Extra Vitamins and Minerals Help?

Many cancer patients want to know whether vitamins, minerals, or other dietary supplements will help "build them up" or fight their cancer. We know that patients who eat well during cancer treatment are better able to cope with their disease and any side effects of treatment. However, there is no scientific evidence that dietary supplements or herbal remedies can cure cancer or stop it from coming back. Large doses of some vitamins may even prevent your cancer treatment from working the way it should. Too-small doses of vitamins and minerals can be just as dangerous. It's best not to begin taking these products on your own. Talk with your doctor or nurse about vitamins or mineral supplements to figure out what's right for you.

What About Alternative Therapies?

You may hear or read about many different kinds of treatment people have tried to cure their disease. A therapy is called complementary when it is used *in addition to* conventional treatments; it is often called alternative when it is used *instead of* conventional treatment. A number of medical centers are evaluating the scientific aspects of complementary and alternative therapies and developing studies to test them. Many of these treatments have not been thoroughly studied, and we have no proof that they work *or* that they are safe. Other "unconventional" treatments have been studied, and we know already that they don't help or are harmful. It is important to talk with your doctor or nurse if you are considering trying any of these treatments, because some therapies may interfere with your standard treatment; others may be harmful when used with conventional treatment. Your medical team can brief you about research that has been done and whether a treatment is safe or would interfere with your treatment. It is important to follow a treatment program as prescribed by your doctor, who uses accepted and proven methods or treatments. People who depend on unconventional treatments alone may lose valuable treatment time and reduce their chances of controlling their cancer and getting well.

Resources

Information about cancer is available from many sources, including the ones listed here. For additional information, you may wish to check your local library, bookstores, or support groups in your community. The health, science, or local events section of your local newspaper may list cancer support or information resources. The Internet can also be a source of information about cancer and cancer treatment. Check with your health-care team for the most reliable Internet sites for medical information.

Organizations

National Cancer Institute (NCI)
Cancer Information Service (CIS)

The CIS, a national information and education network, is a free public service of the NCI, the nation's primary agency for cancer research. The CIS meets the information needs of patients, the public, and health professionals. Specially trained staff provide the latest scientific information in understandable language. CIS staff answer questions in English and Spanish and distribute NCI materials. To reach the CIS, call the toll-free phone number: 1-800-4-CANCER (1-800-422-6237). TTY: 1-800-332-8615.

American Dietetic Association (ADA)

The ADA is a professional society of registered dietitians and other professionals working in food and nutrition-related fields. For a referral to a registered dietitian in your area and to listen to recorded food and nutrition messages, call the ADA's consumer nutrition hotline at 1-800-366-1655. Or visit the ADA's home page on the World Wide Web at http://www.eatright.org.

Making This Book Work for You

Quick and Easy Snacks and Meals

One of the special strengths of this collection of Healthy Exchanges recipes is that just about every dish from every category can be prepared quickly, requires a minimum of work in the kitchen, and is designed to be flavor-rich and high in eye appeal. Of course, not every recipe will appeal to every reader, so you might want to begin by paging through the book and making a list of those dishes that sound good and contain ingredients you like. You'll see that JoAnna's recipes usually serve four to six people, so you'll have tasty leftovers to refrigerate and freeze for another time.

If you don't have a set of handy plastic containers in several sizes, I recommend investing in one. Being able to open the refrigerator and choose something ready-made and good for you is a big help during those times when you don't have the energy or inclination to prepare something.

How to Increase Calories

If your goal during and after cancer treatment is to increase calories, here are some suggestions for using this cookbook:

- Pay attention to portion sizes. Often, the suggested serving size of one of JoAnna's sweet salads or main dishes is less than the amount you might choose to eat. Go for it! Have three-quarters of a cup instead of a half cup, or if you find a recipe especially appealing, why not double the serving and enjoy every bite? On the other hand, if you're not feeling all that hungry, or not able to eat very much on a given day, choose calorie-rich foods that give you lots of "bang for the buck."

- Substitute "the real thing" for low-fat and low-sugar ingredients. Instead of using reduced-fat shredded cheeses, choose the standard version. The same is true for products like sour cream, cottage cheese, and even JELL-O puddings. Healthy Exchanges recipes are particularly useful for weight loss and maintenance, but if you need more calories in your diet, try adjusting the ingredients to suit your needs.

How to Increase Protein

In recent years, most Americans have tried to reduce the amount of protein in their daily menus, since nutritional studies suggested they were overeating this nutrient. But during your treatment and recovery, your medical team may ask you to increase the protein you consume to aid in your return to good health. Since every Healthy Exchanges recipe provides nutrition information, including protein grams, you can create menus that are as high in protein as they are rich in taste appeal. Look for main dishes where you get at least 16 to 20 grams of protein per serving, like Baked Fish with Corn Salsa (24 grams!) or Diane's Angel Hair Pasta and Chicken (26 grams!). Remember that milk products are also good protein sources, so you can enjoy a slice of Easy Pumpkin Raisin Pie and know you're getting 9 grams of protein just with your dessert.

Can You Do Anything to Prevent Cancer?

It seems that every week we open the newspaper to read about a new study, either about what foods may give us cancer, or what foods may keep us from getting it. I've discussed this concern with medical professionals and tried to keep an open mind on the subject. Ultimately, I think what we know is this: certain behaviors and certain foods appear to improve our chances of getting and staying healthy. If we can keep our immune systems strong, our bodies will do their best to protect us. There are no guarantees, of course, but I think it's a smart decision to do the best you can. Here are some recommendations, developed from the medical advice I've received and the many articles and books I've read:

- Don't smoke. If you do, get help so you can stop. This is one risk factor we're sure about.

- Limit alcohol. Research suggests that the more alcohol you consume, the greater your chance of getting cancer of the colon, mouth, and liver. You don't have to be a teetotaler, but keep my watchword "Moderation" in mind.

- Eat a low-fat diet that emphasizes fruits, veggies, legumes, and complex carbohydrates. Why do we like these foods? They're high in fiber, vitamins, minerals, and those cancer-fighting agents, antioxidants. Government recommendations want you to have "five a day" of fruits and vegetables. Leafy green vegetables and citrus fruits are especially good for lowering your risk of certain cancers—breast, stomach, lung, colon, and bladder among them. The "good things" in fruits and veggies include beta-carotene, vitamin C, vitamin E, and selenium. Very recent studies encourage us to eat tomatoes for their lycopene and carrots for carotenoids, both of which appear to help in the fight against cancer. Other studies push the "cruciferous" vegetables like broccoli, cauliflower, and cabbage, while still others celebrate the cancer-protective qualities of onions and garlic.

The other firm recommendation is to boost complex carbohydrates by eating "seven a day" of whole grains and root veggies, so enjoy your rice, sweet potatoes, beets, and turnips, all the while knowing that you are doing good while eating well.

- Avoid gaining weight as you get older. Weight gain has been linked to increased cancer risks.

Some other suggestions from various sources: limit salt, drink black or green tea, add soy foods to your menus, and avoid eating foods that have been overly blackened by charcoal grilling.

It sounds like a lot to think about, but don't stress yourself out! Too much stress can be as dangerous to your good health as eating unhealthy foods. Find outlets that help you relieve stress and handle the day-to-day demands of your busy life. These include moderate exercise, relaxing activities and hobbies, and perhaps most important, daily contact with friends and people who care about you.

Here's to your good health!

Dear Friends,

People often ask me why I include the same general information at the beginning of all my cookbooks. If you've seen any of my other books you'll know that my "common folk" recipes are just one part of the Healthy Exchanges picture. You know that I firmly believe—and say so whenever and wherever I can— that *Healthy Exchanges is not a diet, it's a way of life!* That's why I include the story of Healthy Exchanges in every book, because I know that the tale of my struggle to lose weight and regain my health is one that speaks to the hearts of many thousands of people. And because Healthy Exchanges is not just a collection of recipes, I always include the wisdom that I've learned from my own experiences and the knowledge of the health and cooking professionals I meet. Whether it's learning about nutrition or making shopping and cooking easier, no Healthy Exchanges book would be complete without features like "A Peek into My Pantry" or "JoAnna's Ten Commandments of Successful Cooking."

Even if you've read my other books, you might still want to skim the following chapters—you never know when I'll slip in a new bit of wisdom or suggest a new product that will make your journey to health an easier and tastier one. If you're sharing this book with a friend or family member, you'll want to make sure they read the following pages before they start stirring up the recipes.

If this is the first book of mine that you've read, I want to welcome you with all my heart to the Healthy Exchanges Family. (And, of course, I'd love to hear your comments or questions. See the back of the book for my mailing address.)

Jo Anna

JoAnna M. Lund

and Healthy

Exchanges

Food is the first invited guest to every special occasion in every family's memory scrapbook. From baptism to graduation, from bar mitzvahs to anniversaries, and from weddings to wakes, food brings us together.

It wasn't always that way at our house. I used to eat alone, even when my family was there, because while they were dining on real food, I was nibbling at whatever my newest diet called for. In fact, for twenty-eight years, I called myself the diet queen of DeWitt, Iowa.

I tried every diet I ever came across, every one I could afford, and every one that found its way to my small town in eastern Iowa. I was willing to try anything that promised to "melt off the pounds," determined to deprive my body in every possible way in order to become thin at last.

I sent away for expensive "miracle" diet pills. I starved myself on the Cambridge Diet and the Bahama Diet. I gobbled diet candies, took thyroid pills, fiber pills, prescription and over-the-counter diet pills. I went to endless weight-loss support group meetings—but I somehow managed to turn healthy programs such as Over-eaters Anonymous, Weight Watchers, and TOPS into unhealthy diets . . . diets I could never follow for more than a few months.

I was determined to discover something that worked long-term, but each new failure increased my desperation that I'd never find it.

I ate strange concoctions and rubbed on even stranger potions. I tried liquid diets. I agreed to be hypnotized. I tried reflexology and even had an acupressure device stuck in my ear!

Does my story sound a lot like yours? I'm not surprised. No wonder the weight-loss business is a billion-dollar industry!

Every new thing I tried seemed to work—at least at first. And losing that first five or ten pounds would get me so excited, I'd believe that this new miracle diet would, finally, get my weight off for keeps.

Inevitably, though, the initial excitement wore off. The diet's routine and boredom set in, and I quit. I shoved the pills to the back of the medicine chest; pushed the cans of powdered shake mix to the rear of the kitchen cabinets; slid all the program materials out of sight under my bed; and once more I felt like a failure.

Like most dieters, I quickly gained back the weight I'd lost each time, along with a few extra "souvenir" pounds that seemed always to settle around my hips. I'd done the diet-lose-weight-gain-it-all-back "yo-yo" on the average of once a year. It's no exaggeration to say that over the years I've lost 1,000 pounds—and gained back 1,150 pounds.

Finally, at the age of forty-six I weighed more than I'd ever imagined possible. I'd stopped believing that any diet could work for me. I drowned my sorrows in sacks of cake donuts and wondered if I'd live long enough to watch my grandchildren grow up.

Something had to change.

I had to change.

Finally, I did.

I'm over fifty now—and I'm 130 pounds less than my all-time high of close to 300 pounds. I've kept the weight off for more than seven years. I'd like to lose another ten pounds, but I'm not obsessed about it. If it takes me two or three years to accomplish it, that's okay.

What I *do* care about is never saying hello again to any of those unwanted pounds I said good-bye to!

How did I jump off the roller coaster I was on? For one thing, I finally stopped looking to food to solve my emotional problems. But what really shook me up—and got me started on the path that changed my life—was Operation Desert Storm in early 1991. I sent three children off to the Persian Gulf War—my son-in-law, Matt, a medic in Special Forces; my daughter, Becky, a full-time college student and member of a medical unit in the Army Reserve; and my son, James, a member of the Inactive Army Reserve reactivated as a chemicals expert.

Somehow, knowing that my children were putting their lives on the line got me thinking about my own mortality—and I knew in my heart the last thing they needed while they were overseas was to get a letter from home saying that their mother was ill because of a food-related problem.

The day I drove the third child to the airport to leave for Saudi Arabia, something happened to me that would change my life for the better—and forever. I stopped praying my constant prayer as a professional dieter, which was simply "Please, God, let me lose ten pounds by Friday." Instead, I began praying, "God, please help me not to be a burden to my kids and my family." I quit praying for what I wanted and started praying for what I needed—and in the process my prayers were answered. I couldn't keep the kids safe—that was out of my hands—but I could try to get healthier to better handle the stress of it. It was the least I could do on the homefront.

That quiet prayer was the beginning of the new JoAnna Lund. My initial goal was not to lose weight or create healthy recipes. I only wanted to become healthier for my kids, my husband, and myself.

Each of my children returned safely from the Persian Gulf War. But something didn't come back—the 130 extra pounds I'd been lugging around for far too long. I'd finally accepted the truth after all those agonizing years of suffering through on-again, off-again dieting.

There are no "magic" cures in life.

No "miracle" potion, pill, or diet will make unwanted pounds disappear.

I found something better than magic, if you can believe it. When I turned my weight and health dilemma over to God for guidance, a new JoAnna Lund and Healthy Exchanges were born.

I discovered a new way to live my life—and uncovered an unexpected talent for creating easy "common folk" healthy recipes, and sharing my commonsense approach to healthy living. I learned that I could motivate others to change their lives and adopt a positive outlook. I began publishing cookbooks and a monthly food newsletter, and speaking to groups all over the country.

I like to say, *"When life handed me a lemon, not only did I make healthy, tasty lemonade, I wrote the recipe down!"*

What I finally found was not a quick fix or a short-term diet, but a great way to live well for a lifetime.

I want to share it with you.

Food Exchanges

and Weight

Loss Choices™

While many people recovering from cancer are not primarily interested in losing weight, the Healthy Exchanges recipes in this book can be used as part of a healthy eating plan and to assist in weight loss. For that reason, I have included general information about using the Exchange system that has helped me and others lose weight.

If you've ever been on one of the national weight-loss programs like Weight Watchers or Diet Center, you've already been introduced to the concept of measured portions of different food groups that make up your daily food plan. If you are not familiar with such a system of weight-loss choices or exchanges, here's a brief explanation. (If you want or need more detailed information, you can write to the American Dietetic Association or the American Diabetes Association for comprehensive explanations.)

The idea of food exchanges is to divide foods into basic food groups. The foods in each group are measured in servings that have comparable values. These groups include Proteins/Meats, Breads/Starches, Fruits, Skim Milk, Vegetables, Fats, Free Foods, and Optional Calories.

Each choice or exchange included in a particular group has about the same number of calories and a similar carbohydrate, protein, and fat content as the other foods in that group. Because any food on a particular list can be "exchanged" for any other food in that group, it makes sense to call the food groups *exchanges* or *choices.*

I like to think we are also "exchanging" bad habits and food choices for good ones!

By using Weight Loss Choices or exchanges you can choose from a variety of foods without having to calculate the nutrient value of each one. This makes it easier to include a wide variety of foods in your daily menus and gives you the opportunity to tailor your choices to your unique appetite.

If you want to lose weight, you should consult your physician or other weight-control expert regarding the number of servings that would be best for you from each food group. Since men generally require more calories than women, and since the requirements for growing children and teenagers differ from those of adults, the right number of exchanges for any one person is a personal decision.

I have included a suggested plan of weight-loss choices in the pages following the exchange lists. It's a program I used to lose 130 pounds, and it's the one I still follow today.

(If you are a diabetic or have been diagnosed with heart problems, it is best to meet with your physician before using this or any other food program or recipe collection.)

Food Group Weight Loss Choices/Exchanges

Not all food group exchanges are alike. The ones that follow are for anyone who's interested in weight loss or maintenance. If you are a diabetic, you should check with your health-care provider or dietitian to get the information you need to help you plan your diet. Diabetic exchanges are calculated by the American Diabetic Association, and information about them is provided in *The Diabetic's Healthy Exchanges Cookbook* (Perigee Books).

Every Healthy Exchanges recipe provides calculations in three ways:

- Weight Loss Choices / Exchanges

- Calories, Fat, Protein, Carbohydrates, and Fiber in grams, and Sodium and Calcium in milligrams

- Diabetic Exchanges calculated for me by a registered dietitian

Healthy Exchanges recipes can help you eat well and recover your health, whatever your health concerns may be. Please take a few minutes to review the exchange lists and the suggestions that follow on how to count them. You have lots of great eating in store for you!

Proteins / Meats

Meat, poultry, seafood, eggs, cheese, and legumes. One exchange of Protein is approximately 60 calories. Examples of one Protein choice or exchange:

1 ounce cooked weight of lean meat, poultry, or seafood
2 ounces white fish
1½ ounces 97% fat-free ham
1 egg (limit to no more than 4 per week)
¼ cup egg substitute
3 egg whites
¾ ounce reduced-fat cheese
½ cup fat-free cottage cheese
2 ounces cooked or ¾ ounce uncooked dry beans
1 tablespoon peanut butter (also count 1 fat exchange)

Breads / Starches

Breads, crackers, cereals, grains, and starchy vegetables. One exchange of Bread is approximately 80 calories. Examples of one Bread choice or exchange:

1 slice bread or 2 slices reduced-calorie bread (40 calories or less)
1 roll, any type (1 ounce)
½ cup cooked pasta or ¾ ounce uncooked (scant ½ cup)
½ cup cooked rice or 1 ounce uncooked (⅓ cup)

3 tablespoons flour
3/4 ounce cold cereal
1/2 cup cooked hot cereal or 3/4 ounce uncooked (2 tablespoons)
1/2 cup corn (kernels or cream style) or peas
4 ounces white potato, cooked, or 5 ounces uncooked
3 ounces sweet potato, cooked, or 4 ounces uncooked
3 cups air-popped popcorn
7 fat-free crackers (3/4 ounce)
3 (2 1/2-inch squares) graham crackers
2 (3/4-ounce) rice cakes or 6 mini rice cakes
1 tortilla, any type (6-inch diameter)

Fruits

All fruits and fruit juices. One exchange of Fruit is approximately
60 calories. Examples of one Fruit choice or exchange:

1 small apple or 1/2 cup slices
1 small orange
1/2 medium banana
3/4 cup berries (except strawberries and cranberries)
1 cup strawberries or cranberries
1/2 cup canned fruit, packed in fruit juice or rinsed well
2 tablespoons raisins
1 tablespoon spreadable fruit spread
1/2 cup apple juice (4 fluid ounces)
1/2 cup orange juice (4 fluid ounces)
1/2 cup applesauce

Skim Milk

Milk, buttermilk, and yogurt. One exchange of Skim Milk is
approximately 90 calories. Examples of one Skim Milk choice or
exchange:

1 cup skim milk
1/2 cup evaporated skim milk
1 cup low-fat buttermilk
3/4 cup plain fat-free yogurt
1/3 cup nonfat dry milk powder

Vegetables

All fresh, canned, or frozen vegetables other than the starchy vegetables. One exchange of Vegetable is approximately 30 calories. Examples of one Vegetable choice or exchange:

> ½ cup vegetable
> ¼ cup tomato sauce
> 1 medium fresh tomato
> ½ cup vegetable juice

Fats

Margarine, mayonnaise, vegetable oils, salad dressings, olives, and nuts. One exchange of Fat is approximately 40 calories. Examples of one Fat choice or exchange:

> 1 teaspoon margarine or 2 teaspoons reduced-calorie margarine
> 1 teaspoon butter
> 1 teaspoon vegetable oil
> 1 teaspoon mayonnaise or 2 teaspoons reduced-calorie mayonnaise
> 1 teaspoon peanut butter
> 1 ounce olives
> ¼ ounce pecans or walnuts

Free Foods

Foods that do not provide nutritional value but are used to enhance the taste of foods are included in the Free Foods group. Examples of these are spices, herbs, extracts, vinegar, lemon juice, mustard, Worcestershire sauce, and soy sauce. Cooking sprays and artificial sweeteners used in moderation are also included in this group. However, you'll see that I include the caloric value of artificial sweeteners in the Optional Calories of the recipes.

You may occasionally see a recipe that lists "free food" as part of the portion. According to the published exchange lists, a free food contains fewer than 20 calories per serving. Two or three servings per day of free foods/drinks are usually allowed in a meal plan.

Optional Calories

Foods that do not fit into any other group but are used in moderation in recipes are included in Optional Calories. Foods that are counted in this way include sugar-free gelatin and puddings, fat-free mayonnaise and dressings, reduced-calorie whipped toppings, reduced-calorie syrups and jams, chocolate chips, coconut, and canned broth.

Sliders™

These are 80 Optional Calorie increments that do not fit into any particular category. You can choose which food group to *slide* these into. It is wise to limit this selection to approximately three to four per day to ensure the best possible nutrition for your body while still enjoying an occasional treat.

Sliders may be used in either of the following ways:

1. If you have consumed all your Protein, Bread, Fruit, or Skim Milk Weight Loss Choices for the day, and you want to eat additional foods from those food groups, you simply use a Slider. It's what I call "healthy horse trading." Remember that Sliders may not be traded for choices in the Vegetables or Fats food groups.

2. Sliders may also be deducted from your Optional Calories for the day or week. One-quarter Slider equals 20 Optional Calories; ½ Slider equals 40 Optional Calories; ¾ Slider equals 60 Optional Calories; and 1 Slider equals 80 Optional Calories.

Healthy Exchanges Weight Loss Choices

My original Healthy Exchanges program of Weight Loss Choices was based on an average daily total of 1,400 to 1,600 calories per day. That was what I determined was right for my needs, and for those of most women. Because men require additional calories (about 1,600 to 1,900), here are my suggested plans for women and men. (*If you require more or fewer calories, please revise this plan to meet your individual needs.*)

Each day, women should plan to eat:

2 Skim Milk choices, 90 calories each
2 Fat choices, 40 calories each
3 Fruit choices, 60 calories each
4 Vegetable choices or more, 30 calories each
5 Protein choices, 60 calories each
5 Bread choices, 80 calories each

Each day, men should plan to eat:

2 Skim Milk choices, 90 calories each
4 Fat choices, 40 calories each
3 Fruit choices, 60 calories each
4 Vegetable choices or more, 30 calories each
6 Protein choices, 60 calories each
7 Bread choices, 80 calories each

Young people should follow the program for men but add 1 Skim Milk choice for a total of 3 servings.

You may also choose to add up to 100 Optional Calories per day, and up to 21 to 28 Sliders per week at 80 calories each. If you choose to include more Sliders in your daily or weekly totals, deduct those 80 calories from your Optional Calorie "bank."

A word about **Sliders:** These are to be counted toward your totals after you have used your allotment of choices of Skim Milk, Protein, Bread, and Fruit for the day. By "sliding" an additional choice into one of these groups, you can meet your individual needs for that day. Sliders are especially helpful when traveling, stressed-out, eating out, or for special events. I often use mine so I can enjoy my favorite Healthy Exchanges desserts. Vegetables are not to be counted as Sliders. Enjoy as many Vegetable choices as you need to feel satisfied. Because we want to limit our fat intake to moderate amounts, additional Fat choices should not be counted as Sliders. If you choose to include more fat on an *occasional* basis, count the extra choices as Optional Calories.

Keep a daily food diary of your Weight Loss Choices, checking off what you eat as you go. If, at the end of the day, your required selections are not 100 percent accounted for, but you have done the best you can, go to bed with a clear conscience. There will be days when you have ¼ Fruit or ½ Bread left over. What are you going to do—eat two slices of an orange or half a slice of bread and throw the rest out? I always say, "Nothing in life comes out exact." Just do the best you can . . . *the best you can.*

Try to drink at least eight 8-ounce glasses of water a day. Water truly is the "nectar" of good health.

As a little added insurance, I take a multivitamin each day. It's not essential, but if my day's worth of well-planned meals "bites the dust" when unexpected events intrude on my regular routine, my body still gets its vital nutrients.

The calories listed in each group of choices are averages. Some choices within each group may be higher or lower, so it's important to select a variety of different foods instead of eating the same three or four all the time.

Use your Optional Calories! They are what I call "life's little extras." They make all the difference in how you enjoy your food and appreciate the variety available to you. Yes, we can get by without them, but do you really want to? Keep in mind that you should be using all your daily Weight Loss Choices first to ensure you are getting the basics of good nutrition. But I guarantee that Optional Calories will keep you from feeling deprived—and help you reach your weight-loss goals.

Sodium, Fat, Cholesterol, and Processed Foods

*A*re Healthy Exchanges *ingredients really healthy?*
When I first created Healthy Exchanges, many people asked about sodium, about whether it was necessary to calculate the percentage of fat, saturated fat, and cholesterol in a healthy diet, and about my use of processed foods in many recipes. I researched these questions as I was developing my program, so you can feel confident about using the recipes and food plan.

Sodium

Most people consume more sodium than their bodies need. The American Heart Association and the American Diabetes Association recommend limiting daily sodium intake to no more than 3,000 milligrams per day. If your doctor suggests you limit your sodium even more, then *you really must read labels.*

Sodium is an essential nutrient and should not be completely eliminated. It helps to regulate blood volume and is needed for normal daily muscle and nerve functions. Most of us, however, have no trouble getting "all we need" and then some.

As with everything else, moderation is my approach. I rarely ever have salt on my list as an added ingredient. But if you're especially sodium-sensitive, make the right choices for you—and save high-sodium foods such as sauerkraut for an occasional treat.

I use lots of spices to enhance flavors, so you won't notice the absence of salt. In the few cases where it is used, salt is vital for the success of the recipe, so please don't omit it.

When I do use an ingredient high in sodium, I try to compensate by using low-sodium products in the remainder of the recipe. Many fat-free products are a little higher in sodium to make up for any loss of flavor that disappeared along with the fat. But when I take advantage of these fat-free, higher-sodium products, I stretch that ingredient within the recipe, lowering the amount of sodium per serving. A good example is my use of fat-free and reduced-sodium canned soups. While the suggested number of servings per can is two, I make sure my final creation serves at least four and sometimes six. So the soup's sodium has been "watered down" from one-third to one-half of the original amount.

Even if you don't have to watch your sodium intake for medical reasons, using moderation is another "healthy exchange" to make on your own journey to good health.

Fat Percentages

We've been told that 30 percent is the magic number—that we should limit fat intake to 30 percent or less of our total calories. It's good advice, and I try to have a weekly average of 15 percent to 25 percent myself. I believe any less than 15 percent is really just another restrictive diet that won't last. And more than 25 percent on a regular basis is too much of a good thing.

When I started listing fat grams along with calories in my recipes, I was tempted to include the percentage of calories from fat. After all, in the vast majority of my recipes, that percentage is well below 30 percent This even includes my pie recipes that allow you a realistic serving instead of many "diet" recipes that tell you a serving is 1/12 of a pie.

Figuring fat grams is easy enough. Each gram of fat equals 9 calories. Multiply fat grams by 9, then divide that number by the total calories to get the percentage of calories from fat.

So why don't I do it? After consulting four registered dietitians for advice, I decided to omit this information. They felt that it's too easy for people to become obsessed by that 30 percent figure, which is after all supposed to be a percentage of total calories over the course of a day or a week. We mustn't feel we can't include a healthy ingredient such as pecans or olives in one recipe just because, on its own, it has more than 30 percent of its calories from fat.

An example of this would be a casserole made with 90 percent lean red meat. Most of us benefit from eating red meat in moderation, as it provides iron and niacin in our diets, and it also makes life more enjoyable for us and those who eat with us. If we *only* look at the percentage of calories from fat in a serving of this one dish, which might be as high as 40 to 45 percent, we might choose not to include this recipe in our weekly food plan.

The dietitians suggested that it's important to consider the total picture when making such decisions. As long as your overall food plan keeps fat calories to 30 percent, it's all right to enjoy an occasional dish that is somewhat higher in fat content. Healthy foods I include in **MODERATION** include 90 percent lean red meat, olives, and nuts. I don't eat these foods every day, and you may not either. But occasionally, in a good recipe, they make all the difference in the world between just getting by (deprivation) and truly enjoying your food.

Remember, the goal is eating in a healthy way so you can enjoy and live well the rest of your life.

Saturated Fats and Cholesterol

You'll see that I don't provide calculations for saturated fats or cholesterol amounts in my recipes. It's for the simple and yet not so simple reason that accurate, up-to-date, brand-specific information can be difficult to obtain from food manufacturers, especially since the way in which they produce food keeps changing rapidly. But once more I've consulted with registered dietitians and other professionals and found that, because I use only a few products that are high in saturated fat, and use them in such limited quantities, my recipes are suitable for patients concerned about controlling or lowering cholesterol. You'll also find that whenever I do use one of these ingredients *in moderation*, everything else in the recipe, and in the meals my family and I enjoy, is low in fat.

Processed Foods

Just what is processed food, anyway? What do I mean by the term "processed foods," and why do I use them, when the "purest" recipe developers in Recipe Land consider them "pedestrian" and won't ever use something from a box, container, or can? A letter I received and a passing statement from a stranger made me reflect on what I mean when I refer to processed foods, and helped me reaffirm why I use them in my "common folk" healthy recipes.

If you are like the vast millions who agree with me, then I'm not sharing anything new with you. And if you happen to disagree, that's okay, too.

A while back, a woman sent me several articles from various "whole food" publications and wrote that she was wary of processed foods, and wondered why I used them in my recipes. She then scribbled on the bottom of her note, "Just how healthy is Healthy Exchanges?" Then, a few weeks later, during a chance visit at a public food event with a very pleasant woman, I was struck by how we all have our own definitions of what processed foods are. She shared with me, in a somewhat self-righteous manner, that she *never* uses processed foods. She only cooked with fresh fruits and vegetables, she told me. Then later she said that she used canned reduced-fat soups all the time! Was her definition different than mine, I wondered? Soup in a can, whether it's reduced in fat or not, still meets my definition of a processed food.

So I got out a copy of my book *HELP: Healthy Exchanges Lifetime Plan* and reread what I had written back then about processed foods. Nothing in my definition had changed since I wrote that section. I still believe that healthy processed foods, such as canned soups, prepared piecrusts, sugar-free instant puddings, fat-free sour cream, and frozen whipped topping, when used properly, all have a place as ingredients in healthy recipes.

I never use an ingredient that hasn't been approved by either the American Diabetic Association, the American Dietetic Association, or the American Heart Association. Whenever I'm in doubt, I send for their position papers, then ask knowledgeable registered dietitians to explain those papers to me in layman's language. I've been assured by all of them that the sugar- and fat-free products I use in my recipes are indeed safe.

If you don't agree, nothing I can say or write will convince you otherwise. But, if you've been using the healthy processed foods and have been concerned about the almost daily hoopla you hear about yet another product that's going to be the doom of all of us, then just stick with reason. For every product on the grocery shelves, there are those who want you to buy it and there are those who don't, *because they want you to buy their products instead.* So we have to learn to sift the fact from the fiction. Let's take sugar substitutes, for example. In making your own evaluations, you should be skeptical about any information provided by the sugar substitute manufacturers, because they have a vested interest in our buying their products. Likewise, ignore any information provided by the sugar industry, because they have a vested interest in our *not* buying sugar substitutes. Then, if you aren't sure if you can really trust the government or any of its agencies, toss out their data, too. That leaves the three associations I mentioned earlier. Do you think any of them would say a product is safe if it isn't? Or say a product isn't safe when it is? They have nothing to gain or lose, *other than their integrity*, if they intentionally try to mislead us. That's why I only go to these associations for information concerning healthy processed foods.

I certainly don't recommend that everything we eat should come from a can, box, or jar. I think the best of all possible worlds is to start with the basics: grains such as rice, pasta, or corn. Then, for example, add some raw vegetables and extra-lean meat such as poultry, fish, beef, or pork. Stir in some healthy canned soup or tomato sauce, and you'll end up with something that is not only healthy but tastes so good, everyone from toddlers to great-grandparents will want to eat it!

I've never been in favor of spraying everything we eat with chemicals, and I don't believe that all our foods should come out of packages. But I do think we should use the best available healthy processed foods to make cooking easier and food taste better. I take advantage of the good-tasting low-fat and low-sugar products found in any grocery store. My recipes are created for busy people like me, people who want to eat healthily and economically but who still want the food to satisfy their tastebuds. I don't expect anyone to visit out-of-the-way health food stores or find the time to cook beans from scratch—*because I don't!* Most of you can't grow fresh food in the backyard and many of you may not have access to farmers' markets or large supermarkets. I want to help you figure out realistic ways to make healthy eating a reality *wherever you live*, or you will not stick to a healthy lifestyle for long.

So if you've been swayed (by individuals or companies with vested interests or hidden agendas) into thinking that all processed foods are bad for you, you may want to reconsider your position. Or if you've been fooling yourself into believing that you *never* use processed foods but regularly reach for that healthy canned soup, stop playing games with yourself—you are using processed foods in a healthy way. And, if you're like me and use healthy processed foods in *moderation*, don't let anyone make you feel ashamed about including these products in your healthy lifestyle. Only *you* can decide what's best for *you* and your family's needs.

Part of living a healthy lifestyle is making those decisions and then getting on with life. Congratulations on choosing to live a healthy lifestyle, and let's celebrate together by sharing a piece of Healthy Exchanges pie that I've garnished with Cool Whip Lite!

JoAnna's Ten Commandments of Successful Cooking

A very important part of any journey is knowing where you are going and the best way to get there. If you plan and prepare before you start to cook, you should reach mealtime with foods to write home about!

1. **Read the entire recipe from start to finish** and be sure you understand the process involved. Check that you have all the equipment you will need *before* you begin.

2. **Check the ingredient list** and be sure you have *everything* and in the amounts required. Keep cooking sprays handy—while they're not listed as ingredients, I use them all the time (just a quick squirt!).

3. **Set out** *all* the ingredients and equipment needed to prepare the recipe on the counter near you *before* you start. Remember that old saying *A stitch in time saves nine?* It applies in the kitchen, too.

4. **Do as much advance preparation as possible** before actually cooking. Chop, cut, grate, or do whatever is needed to prepare the ingredients and have them ready before you start to mix. Turn the oven on at least ten minutes before putting food in to bake, to allow the oven to preheat to the proper temperature.

5. **Use a kitchen timer** to tell you when the cooking or baking time is up. Because stove temperatures vary slightly by manufacturer, you may want to set your timer for five minutes less than the suggested time just to prevent overcooking. Check the progress of your dish at that time, then decide if you need the additional minutes or not.

6. **Measure carefully.** Use glass measures for liquids and metal or plastic cups for dry ingredients. My recipes are based on standard measurements. Unless I tell you it's a scant or full cup, measure the cup level.

7. **For best results, follow the recipe instructions exactly.** Feel free to substitute ingredients that *don't tamper* with the basic chemistry of the recipe, but be sure to leave key ingredients alone. For example, you could substitute sugar-free instant chocolate pudding for sugar-free instant butterscotch pudding, but if you use a six-serving package when a four-serving package was listed in the ingredients, or you use instant when cook-and-serve is required, you won't get the right result.

8. **Clean up as you go.** It is much easier to wash a few items at a time than to face a whole counter of dirty dishes later. The same is true for spills on the counter or floor.

9. **Be careful about doubling or halving a recipe.** Though many recipes can be altered successfully to serve more or fewer people, *many cannot.* This is especially true when it comes to spices and liquids. If you try to double a recipe that calls for 1 teaspoon pumpkin pie spice, for example, and you double the spice, you may end up with a too-spicy taste. I usually suggest increasing spices or liquid by 1½ times when doubling a recipe. If it tastes a little bland to you, you can increase the spice to 1¾ times the original amount the next time you prepare the dish. Remember: You can always add more, but you can't take it out after it's stirred in.

   The same is true with liquid ingredients. If you wanted to **triple** a recipe like my **Enchilada Casserole** because you were planning to serve a crowd, you might think you should use three times as much of every ingredient. Don't, or you could end up with Enchilada Casserole Soup! The original recipe calls for 1¾ cups of chunky tomato sauce, so I'd suggest using 3½ cups when you **triple** the recipe (or 2¾ cups if you **double** it). You'll still have a good-tasting dish that won't run all over the plate.

10. **Write your reactions next to each recipe once you've served it.** Yes, that's right, I'm giving you permission to write in this book. It's yours, after all. Ask yourself: Did everyone like it? Did you have to add another half teaspoon of chili seasoning to please your family, who like to live on the spicier side of the street? You may even want to rate the recipe on a scale of 1★ to 4★, depending on what you thought of it. (Four stars would be the top rating—and I hope you'll feel that way about many of my recipes.) Jotting down your comments while they are fresh in your mind will help you personalize the recipe to your own taste the next time you prepare it.

My Best Healthy Exchanges Tips and Tidbits

Measurements, General Cooking Tips, and Basic Ingredients

The word **moderation** best describes **my use of fats, sugar substitutes,** and **sodium** in these recipes. Wherever possible, I've used cooking spray for sautéing and for browning meats and vegetables. I also use reduced-calorie margarine and fat-free mayonnaise and salad dressings. Lean ground turkey *or* ground beef can be used in the recipes. Just be sure whatever you choose is at least *90 percent lean.*

Sugar Substitutes

I've also included **small amounts of sugar substitutes as the sweetening agent** in many of the recipes. I don't drink a hundred cans of soda a day or eat enough artificially sweetened foods in a 24-hour time period to be troubled by sugar substitutes. But if this is a concern of yours and you *do not* need to watch your sugar intake, you can always replace the sugar substitutes with processed sugar and the sugar-free products with regular ones.

I created my recipes knowing they would also be used by hypoglycemics, diabetics, and those concerned about triglycerides. If you choose to use sugar instead, be sure to count the additional calories.

A word of caution when cooking with **sugar substitutes**: Use **saccharin**-based sweeteners when **heating or baking**. In recipes that **don't require heat, aspartame** (known as NutraSweet) works well in uncooked dishes but leaves an after-taste in baked products.

Sugar Twin is my first choice for a sugar substitute. If you can't find that, use **Sprinkle Sweet**. They measure like sugar, you can cook and bake with them, they're inexpensive, and they are easily poured from their boxes.

Many of my recipes for quick breads, muffins, and cakes include a package of sugar-free instant pudding mix, which is sweetened with NutraSweet. Yet we've been told that NutraSweet breaks down under heat. I've tested my recipes again and again, and here's what I've found: baking with a NutraSweet product sold for home sweetening doesn't work, but baking with NutraSweet-sweetened instant pudding mixes turns out great. I choose not to question why this is, but continue to use these products in creating my Healthy Exchanges recipes.

How much sweetener is the right amount? I use pourable Sugar Twin, Brown Sugar Twin, and Sprinkle Sweet in my recipes because they measure just like sugar. What could be easier? I also use them because they work wonderfully in cooked and baked products.

If you are using a brand other than these, you need to check the package to figure out how much of your sweetener will equal what's called for in the recipe.

If you choose to use real sugar or brown sugar, then you would use the same amount the recipe lists for pourable Sugar Twin or Brown Sugar Twin.

You'll see that I list only the specific brands when the recipe preparation involves heat. In a salad or other recipe that doesn't require cooking, I will list the ingredient as "sugar substitute to equal 2 tablespoons sugar." You can then use any sweetener you choose—Equal, Sweet 'n Low, Sweet Ten, or any other aspartame-based sugar substitute. Just check the label so you'll be using the right amount to equal those 2 tablespoons of sugar. Or, if you choose, you can use regular sugar.

With Healthy Exchanges recipes, the "sweet life" is the only life for me!

Pan Sizes

I'm often asked why I use an **8-by-8-inch baking dish** in my recipes. It's for portion control. If the recipe says it serves 4, just cut down the center, turn the dish, and cut again. Like magic, there's your serving. Also, if this is the only recipe you are preparing requiring an oven, the square dish fits into a tabletop toaster oven easily and energy can be conserved.

While many of my recipes call for an 8-by-8-inch baking dish, others ask for a 9-by-9-inch cake pan. If you don't have a 9-inch-square pan, is it all right to use your 8-inch dish instead? In most cases, the small difference in the size of these two pans won't significantly affect the finished product, so until you can get your hands on the right size pan, go ahead and use your baking dish.

However, since the 8-inch dish is usually made of glass, and the 9-inch cake pan is made of metal, you will want to adjust the baking temperature. If you're using a glass baking dish in a recipe that calls for a 9-inch pan, be sure to lower your baking temperature by 15 degrees *or* check your finished product at least 6 to 8 minutes before the specified baking time is over.

But it really is worthwhile to add a 9-by-9-inch pan to your collection, and if you're going to be baking lots of my Healthy Exchanges cakes, you'll definitely use it frequently. A cake baked in this pan will have a better texture, and the servings will be a little larger. Just think of it—an 8-by-8-inch pan produces 64 square inches of dessert, while a 9-by-9-inch pan delivers 81 square inches. Those 17 extra inches are too tasty to lose!

To make life even easier, **whenever a recipe calls for ounce measurements** (other than raw meats) I've included the closest cup equivalent. I need to use my scale daily when creating recipes, so I've measured for you at the same time.

Freezing Leftovers

Most of the recipes are for **4 to 8 servings.** If you don't have that many to feed, do what I do: freeze individual portions. Then all you have to do is choose something from the freezer and take it to work for lunch or have your evening meals prepared in advance for the week. In this way, I always have something on hand that is both good to eat and good for me.

Unless a recipe includes hard-boiled eggs, cream cheese, mayonnaise, or a raw vegetable or fruit, **the leftovers should freeze well**. (I've marked recipes that freeze well with the symbol of a **snowflake** ❄.)This includes most of the cream pies. Divide any recipe up into individual servings and freeze for your own "TV" dinners.

Another good idea is **cutting leftover pie into individual pieces and freezing each one separately** in a small Ziploc freezer bag. Once you've cut the pie into portions, place them on a cookie sheet and put it in the freezer for 15 minutes. That way, the creamy topping won't get smashed and your pie will keep its shape.

When you want to thaw a piece of pie for yourself, you don't have to thaw the whole pie. You can practice portion control at the same time, and it works really well for brown-bag lunches. Just pull a piece out of the freezer on your way to work and by lunchtime you will have a wonderful dessert waiting for you.

Why do I so often recommend freezing leftover desserts? One reason is that if you leave baked goods made with sugar substitute out on the counter for more than a day or two, they get moldy. Sugar is a preservative and retards the molding process. It's actually what's called an antimicrobial agent, meaning it works against microbes such as molds, bacteria, fungi, and yeasts that grow in foods and can cause food poisoning. Both sugar and salt work as antimicrobial agents to withdraw water from food. Since microbes can't grow without water, food protected in this way doesn't spoil.

So what do we do if we don't want our muffins to turn moldy, but we also don't want to use sugar because of the excess carbohydrates and calories? Freeze them! Just place each muffin or individually sliced bread serving into a Ziploc sandwich bag, seal, and toss into your freezer. Then, whenever you want one for a snack or a meal, you can choose to let it thaw naturally or "zap" it in the microwave. If you know that baked goods will be eaten within a day or two, packaging them in a sealed plastic container and storing in the refrigerator will do the trick.

Unless I specify **"covered" for simmering or baking**, prepare my recipes **uncovered**. Occasionally you will read a recipe that asks you to cover a dish for a time, then to uncover, so read the directions carefully to avoid confusion—and to get the best results.

Cooking Spray

Low-fat cooking spray is another blessing in a Healthy Exchanges kitchen. It's currently available in three flavors . . .

- **OLIVE OIL FLAVORED** when cooking Mexican, Italian, or Greek dishes

- **BUTTER FLAVORED** when the hint of butter is desired

- **REGULAR** for everything else.

A quick spray of butter-flavored makes air-popped popcorn a low-fat taste treat, or try it as a butter substitute on steaming hot corn on the cob. One light spray of the skillet when browning meat will convince you that you're using "old-fashioned fat," and a quick coating of the casserole dish before you add the ingredients will make serving easier and cleanup quicker.

Baking Times

Sometimes I give you a range as a **baking time**, such as 22 to 28 minutes. Why? Because every kitchen, every stove, and every chef's cooking technique is slightly different. On a hot and humid day in Iowa, the optimum cooking time won't be the same as on a cold, dry day. Some stoves bake hotter than the temperature setting indicates; other stoves bake cooler. Electric ovens usually are more temperamental than gas ovens. If you place your baking pan on a lower shelf, the temperature is warmer than if you place it on a higher shelf. If you stir the mixture more vigorously than I do, you could affect the required baking time by a minute or more.

The best way to gauge the heat of your particular oven is to purchase an oven temperature gauge that hangs in the oven. These can be found in any discount store or kitchen equipment store, and if you're going to be cooking and baking regularly, it's a good idea to own one. Set the oven to 350 degrees and when the oven indicates that it has reached that temperature, check the reading on the gauge. If it's less than 350 degrees, you know your oven cooks cooler, and you need to add a few minutes to the cooking time *or* set your oven at a higher temperature. If it's more than 350 degrees, then your oven is warmer and you need to subtract a few minutes from the cooking time. In any event, always treat the suggested baking time as approximate. Check on your baked product at the earliest suggested time. You can always continue baking a few minutes more if needed, but you can't unbake it once you've cooked it too long.

Miscellaneous Ingredients and Tips

I use reduced-sodium **canned chicken broth** in place of dry bouillon to lower the sodium content. The intended flavor is still present in the prepared dish. As a reduced-sodium beef broth is not currently available (at least not in DeWitt, Iowa), I use the canned regular beef broth. The sodium content is still lower than regular dry bouillon.

Whenever **cooked rice or pasta** is an ingredient, follow the package directions, but eliminate the salt and/or margarine called for. This helps lower the sodium and fat content. It tastes just fine; trust me on this.

Here's another tip: When **cooking rice or noodles**, why not cook extra "for the pot"? After you use what you need, store leftover rice in a covered container (where it will keep for a couple of days). With noodles like spaghetti or macaroni, first rinse and drain as usual, then measure out what you need. Put the leftovers in a bowl covered with water, then store in the refrigerator, covered, until they're needed. Then, measure out what you need, rinse and drain them, and they're ready to go.

Does your **pita bread** often tear before you can make a sandwich? Here's my tip to make them open easily: cut the bread in half, put the halves in the microwave for about 15 seconds, and they will open up by themselves. *Voilà!*

When **chunky salsa** is listed as an ingredient, I leave the degree of "heat" up to your personal taste. In our house, I'm considered a wimp. I go for the "mild" while Cliff prefers "extra-hot." How do we compromise? I prepare the recipe with mild salsa because he can always add a spoonful or two of the hotter version to his serving, but I can't enjoy the dish if it's too spicy for me.

Milk, Yogurt, and More

Take it from me—nonfat dry milk powder is great! I *do not* use it for drinking, but I *do* use it for cooking. Three good reasons why:

1. It is very **inexpensive**.

2. It does not **sour** because you use it only as needed. Store the box in your refrigerator or freezer and it will keep almost forever.

3. You can easily **add extra calcium** to just about any recipe without added liquid.

I consider nonfat dry milk powder one of Mother Nature's modern-day miracles of convenience. But do purchase a good national name brand (I like Carnation), and keep it fresh by proper storage.

I've said many times, "Give me my mixing bowl, my wire whisk, and a box of nonfat dry milk powder, and I can conquer the world!" Here are some of my favorite ways to use dry milk powder:

1. You can make a **pudding** with the nutrients of 2 cups skim milk, but the liquid of only 1¼ to 1½ cups by using ⅔ cup nonfat dry milk powder, a 4-serving package of sugar-free instant pudding, and the lesser amount of water. This makes the pudding taste much creamier and more like homemade. Also, pie filling made my way will set up in minutes. If company is knocking at your door, you can prepare a pie for them almost as fast as you can open the door and invite them in. And if by chance you have left-overs, the filling will not separate the way it does when you use the 2 cups skim milk suggested on the package. (If you absolutely refuse to use this handy powdered milk, you can substitute skim milk in the amount of water I call for. Your pie won't be as creamy, and will likely get runny if you have leftovers.)

2. You can make your own **"sour cream"** by combining ¾ cup plain fat-free yogurt with ⅓ cup nonfat dry milk powder. What you did by doing this is fourfold: (1) The dry milk stabilizes the yogurt and keeps the whey from separating. (2) The dry milk slightly helps to cut the tartness of the yogurt. (3) It's still virtually fat-free. (4) The calcium has been increased by 100 percent. Isn't it great how we can make that distant relative of sour cream a first kissin'

cousin by adding the nonfat dry milk powder? Or, if you place 1 cup plain fat-free yogurt in a sieve lined with a coffee filter, and place the sieve over a small bowl and refrigerate for about 6 hours, you will end up with a very good alternative for sour cream. To **stabilize yogurt** when cooking or baking with it, just add 1 teaspoon cornstarch to every ¾ cup yogurt.

3. You can make **evaporated skim milk** by using ⅓ cup nonfat dry milk powder and ½ cup water for every ½ cup evaporated skim milk you need. This is handy to know when you want to prepare a recipe calling for evaporated skim milk and you don't have any in the cupboard. And if you are using a recipe that requires only 1 cup evaporated skim milk, you don't have to worry about what to do with the leftover milk in the can.

4. You can make **sugar-free and fat-free sweetened condensed milk** by using 1⅓ cups nonfat dry milk powder mixed with ½ cup cold water, microwaved on HIGH until the mixture is hot but not boiling. Then stir in ½ cup Sprinkle Sweet or pourable Sugar Twin. Cover and chill at least 4 hours.

5. For any recipe that calls for **buttermilk**, you might want to try **JO's Buttermilk**: Blend 1 cup water and ⅔ cup nonfat dry milk powder (the nutrients of 2 cups of skim milk). It'll be thicker than this mixed-up milk usually is, because it's doubled. Add 1 teaspoon white vinegar and stir, then let it sit for at least 10 minutes.

What else? Nonfat dry milk powder adds calcium without fuss to many recipes, and it can be stored for months in your refrigerator or freezer.

Soup Substitutes

One of my subscribers was looking for a way to further restrict salt intake and needed a substitute for **cream of mushroom soup**. For many of my recipes, I use Healthy Request Cream of Mushroom Soup, as it is a reduced-sodium product. The label suggests two servings per can, but I usually incorporate the soup into a recipe serving at least four. By doing this, I've reduced the sodium in the soup by half again.

But if you must restrict your sodium even more, try making my Healthy Exchanges **Creamy Mushroom Sauce.** Place 1½ cups evaporated skim milk and 3 tablespoons flour in a covered jar. Shake well and pour the mixture into a medium saucepan sprayed with butter-flavored cooking spray. Add ½ cup canned sliced mushrooms, rinsed and drained. Cook over medium heat, stirring often, until the mixture thickens. Add any seasonings of your choice. You can use this sauce in any recipe that calls for one 10¾-ounce can of cream of mushroom soup.

Why did I choose these proportions and ingredients?

- 1½ cups evaporated skim milk is the amount in one can.

- It's equal to three Skim Milk choices or exchanges.

- It's the perfect amount of liquid and flour for a medium cream sauce.

- 3 tablespoons flour is equal to one bread/starch choice or exchange.

- Any leftovers will reheat beautifully with a flour-based sauce, but not with a cornstarch base.

- The mushrooms are one Vegetable choice or exchange.

- This sauce is virtually fat-free, sugar-free, and sodium-free.

Proteins

Eggs

I use eggs in moderation. I enjoy the real thing on an average of three to four times a week. So, my recipes are calculated on using whole eggs. However, if you choose to use egg substitute in place of the egg, the finished product will turn out just fine and the fat grams per serving will be even lower than those listed.

If you like the look, taste, and feel of **hard-boiled eggs** in salads but haven't been using them because of the cholesterol in the yolk, I have a couple of alternatives for you. (1) Pour an 8-ounce carton of egg substitute into a medium skillet sprayed with cooking spray. Cover the skillet tightly and cook over low heat until substitute is just set, about 10 minutes. Remove from heat and let set, still covered, for 10 minutes more. Uncover and cool completely. Chop the set mixture. This will make about 1 cup of chopped egg. (2) Even easier is to hard-boil "real eggs," toss the yolk away, and chop the white. Either way, you don't deprive yourself of the pleasure of egg in your salad.

In most recipes calling for **egg substitutes**, you can use 2 egg whites in place of the equivalent of 1 egg substitute. Just break the eggs open and toss the yolks away. I can hear some of you already saying, "But that's wasteful!" Well, take a look at the price on the egg substitute package (which usually has the equivalent of 4 eggs in it), then look at the price of a dozen eggs, from which you'd get the equivalent of 6 egg substitutes. Now, what's wasteful about that?

Meats

Whenever I include **cooked chicken** in a recipe, I use roasted white meat without skin. Whenever I include **roast beef or pork** in a recipe, I use the loin cuts because they are much leaner. However, most of the time, I do my roasting of all these meats at the local deli. I just ask for a chunk of their lean roasted meat, 6 or 8 ounces, and ask them not to slice it. When I get home, I cube or dice the meat and am ready to use it in my recipe. The reason I do this is three-fold: (1) I'm getting just the amount I need without leftovers; (2) I don't have the expense of heating the oven; and (3) I'm not throwing away the bone, gristle, and fat I'd be cutting off the meat. Overall, it is probably cheaper to "roast" it the way I do.

Did you know that you can make an acceptable meatloaf without using egg for the binding? Just replace every egg with ¼ cup of liquid. You could use beef broth, tomato sauce, even applesauce, to name just a few. For a meatloaf to serve 6, I always use 1 pound of extra-lean ground beef or turkey, 6 tablespoons of dried fine bread crumbs, and ¼ cup of the liquid, plus anything else healthy that strikes my fancy at the time. I mix well and place the mixture in an 8-by-8-inch baking dish or 9-by-5-inch loaf pan sprayed with cooking spray. Bake uncovered at 350 degrees for 35 to 50 minutes (depending on the added ingredients). You will never miss the egg.

Any time you are **browning ground meat** for a casserole and want to get rid of almost all the excess fat, just place the uncooked meat loosely in a plastic colander. Set the colander in a glass pie plate. Place in the microwave and cook on HIGH for 3 to 6 minutes (depending on the amount being browned), stirring often. Use as you would for any casserole. You can also chop up onions and brown them with the meat if you want.

Gravy

For **gravy** with all the "old time" flavor but without the extra fat, try this almost effortless way to prepare it. (It's almost as easy as opening up a store-bought jar.) Pour the juice off your roasted meat, then set the roast aside to "rest" for about 20 minutes. Place the juice in an uncovered cake pan or other large flat pan (we want the large air surface to speed up the cooling process) and put in the freezer until the fat congeals on top and you can skim it off. Or, if you prefer, use a skimming pitcher purchased at your kitchen gadget store. Either way, measure about 1½ cups skimmed broth and pour into a medium saucepan. Cook over medium heat until heated through, about 5 minutes. In a covered jar, combine ½ cup water or cooled potato broth with 3 tablespoons flour. Shake well. Pour the flour mixture into the warmed juice. Combine well using a wire whisk. Continue cooking until the gravy thickens, about 5 minutes. Season with salt and pepper to taste.

Why did I use flour instead of cornstarch? Because any leftovers will reheat nicely with the flour base and would not with a cornstarch base. Also, 3 tablespoons of flour works out to 1 Bread/Starch exchange. This virtually fat-free gravy makes about 2 cups, so you could spoon about ½ cup gravy on your low-fat mashed potatoes and only have to count your gravy as ¼ Bread/Starch exchange.

Fruits and Vegetables

If you want to enjoy a "**fruit shake**" with some pizzazz, just combine soda water and unsweetened fruit juice in a blender. Add crushed ice. Blend on HIGH until thick. Refreshment without guilt.

You'll see that many recipes use ordinary **canned vegetables.** They're much cheaper than reduced-sodium versions, and once you rinse and drain them, the sodium is reduced anyway. I believe in saving money wherever possible so we can afford the best fat-free and sugar-free products as they come onto the market.

All three kinds of **vegetables—fresh, frozen, and canned—** have their place in a healthy diet. My husband, Cliff, hates the taste of frozen or fresh green beans, thinks the texture is all wrong, so I use canned green beans instead. In this case, canned vegetables have their proper place when I'm feeding my husband. If someone in your family has a similar concern, it's important to respond to it so everyone can be happy and enjoy the meal.

When I use **fruits or vegetables** like apples, cucumbers, and zucchini, I wash them really well and **leave the skin on.** It provides added color, fiber, and attractiveness to any dish. And, because I use processed flour in my cooking, I like to increase the fiber in my diet by eating my fruits and vegetables in their closest-to-natural state.

To help keep **fresh fruits and veggies fresh**, just give them a quick "shower" with lemon juice. The easiest way to do this is to pour purchased lemon juice into a kitchen spray bottle and store in the refrigerator. Then, every time you use fresh fruits or vegetables in a salad or dessert, simply give them a quick spray with your "lemon spritzer." You just might be amazed by how this little trick keeps your produce from turning brown so fast.

The next time you warm canned vegetables such as carrots or green beans, drain and heat the vegetables in ¼ cup beef or chicken broth. It gives a nice variation to an old standby. Here's a simple **white sauce** for vegetables and casseroles, without using added fat, that can be made by spraying a medium saucepan with butter-flavored cooking spray. Place 1½ cups evaporated skim milk and 3 tablespoons flour in a covered jar. Shake well. Pour into the sprayed saucepan and cook over medium heat until thick, stirring constantly. Add salt and pepper to taste. You can also add ½ cup canned drained mushrooms and/or 3 ounces (¾ cup) shredded reduced-fat cheese . Continue cooking until the cheese melts.

Zip up canned or frozen green beans with **chunky salsa**: ½ cup to 2 cups beans. Heat thoroughly. Chunky salsa also makes a wonderful dressing on lettuce salads. It only counts as a vegetable, so enjoy.

Another wonderful **South of the Border** dressing can be stirred up by using ½ cup of chunky salsa and ¼ cup fat-free ranch dressing. Cover and store in your refrigerator. Use as a dressing for salads or as a topping for baked potatoes.

Delightful Dessert Ideas

For a special treat that tastes anything but "diet," try placing **spreadable fruit** in a container and microwave for about 15 seconds. Then pour the melted fruit spread over a serving of nonfat ice cream or frozen yogurt. One tablespoon of spreadable fruit is equal to 1 Fruit choice or exchange. Some combinations to get you started are apricot over chocolate ice cream, strawberry over strawberry ice cream, or any flavor over vanilla.

Another way I use spreadable fruit is to make a delicious **topping for a cheesecake or angel food cake**. I take ½ cup fruit and ½ cup Cool Whip Lite and blend the two together with a teaspoon of coconut extract.

Here's a really **good topping** for fall. Place 1½ cups unsweetened applesauce in a medium saucepan or 4-cup glass measure. Stir in 2 tablespoons raisins, 1 teaspoon apple pie spice, and 2 tablespoons Cary's Sugar Free Maple Syrup. Cook over medium heat on the stovetop or microwave on HIGH until warm. Then spoon about ½ cup of the warm mixture over pancakes, French toast, or sugar- and fat-free vanilla ice cream. It's as close as you will get to guilt-free apple pie!

Do you love hot fudge sundaes as much as I do? Here's my secret for making **Almost Sinless Hot Fudge Sauce.** Just combine the contents of a 4-serving package of JELL-O sugar-free chocolate cook-and-serve pudding with ⅔ cup Carnation Nonfat Dry Milk Powder in a medium saucepan. Add 1¼ cups water. Cook over medium heat, stirring constantly with a wire whisk, until the mixture thickens and starts to boil. Remove from heat and stir in 1 teaspoon vanilla extract, 2 teaspoons reduced-calorie margarine, and ½ cup miniature marshmallows. This makes six ¼-cup servings. Any leftovers can be refrigerated and reheated later in the microwave. Yes, you can buy fat-free chocolate syrup nowadays, but have you checked the sugar content? For a ¼-cup serving of store-bought syrup (and you show me any true hot fudge sundae lover who would settle for less than ¼ cup) it clocks in at over 150 calories with 39 grams of sugar! Hershey's Lite Syrup, while better, still has 100 calories and 10 grams of sugar. But this "homemade" version costs you only 60 calories, less than ½ gram of fat, and just 6 grams of sugar for the same ¼-cup serving. For an occasional squirt on something where 1 teaspoon is enough, I'll use Hershey's Lite Syrup. But when I crave a hot fudge sundae, I scoop out some sugar- and fat-free ice cream, then spoon my Almost Sinless Hot Fudge Sauce over the top and smile with pleasure.

A quick yet tasty way to prepare **strawberries for shortcake** is to place about ¾ cup sliced strawberries, 2 tablespoons Diet Mountain Dew, and sugar substitute to equal ¼ cup sugar in a blender container. Process on BLEND until mixture is smooth. Pour the mixture into bowl. Add 1¼ cups sliced strawberries and mix well. Cover and refrigerate until ready to serve with shortcakes. This tastes just like the strawberry sauce I remember my mother making when I was a child.

Have you tried **thawing Cool Whip Lite** by stirring it? Don't! You'll get a runny mess and ruin the look and taste of your dessert. You can *never* treat Cool Whip Lite the same way you did regular Cool Whip because the "lite" version just doesn't contain enough fat. Thaw your Cool Whip Lite by placing it in your refrigerator at least two hours before you need to use it. When they took the excess fat out of Cool Whip to make it "lite," they replaced it with air. When you stir the living daylights out of it to hurry up the thawing, you also stir out the air. You also can't thaw your Cool Whip Lite in the microwave, or you'll end up with Cool Whip Soup!

Always have a thawed container of Cool Whip Lite in your refrigerator, as it keeps well for up to two weeks. It actually freezes and thaws and freezes and thaws again quite well, so if you won't be using it soon, you could refreeze your leftovers. Just remember to take it out a few hours before you need it, so it'll be creamy and soft and ready to use.

Remember, anytime you see the words "fat-free" or "reduced-fat" on the labels of cream cheese, sour cream, or whipped topping, handle it gently. The fat has been replaced by air or water, and the product has to be treated with special care.

How can you **frost an entire pie with just ½ cup of whipped topping?** First, don't use an inexpensive brand. I use Cool Whip Lite or La Creme Lite. Make sure the topping is fully thawed. Always spread from the center to the sides using a rubber spatula. This way,

½ cup topping will cover an entire pie. Remember, the operative word is *frost,* not pile the entire container on top of the pie!

Another trick I often use is to include tiny amounts of "real people" food, such as coconut, but extend the flavor by using extracts. Try it—you will be surprised by how little of the real thing you can use and still feel you are not being deprived.

If you are preparing a pie filling that has ample moisture, just line the bottom of a 9-by-9-inch cake pan with **graham crackers.** Pour the filling over the top of the crackers. Cover and refrigerate until the moisture has enough time to soften the crackers. Overnight is best. This eliminates the added **fats and sugars of a piecrust.**

One of my readers provided a smart and easy way to enjoy a **two-crust pie** without all the fat that usually comes along with those two crusts. Just use one Pillsbury refrigerated piecrust. Let it set at room temperature for about 20 minutes. Cut the crust in half on the folded line. Gently roll each half into a ball. Wipe your counter with a wet cloth and place a sheet of wax paper on it. Put one of the balls on the wax paper, then cover with another piece of wax paper, and roll it out with your rolling pin. Carefully remove the wax paper on one side and place that side into your 8- or 9-inch pie plate. Fill with your usual pie filling, then repeat the process for the top crust. Bake as usual. Enjoy!

When you are preparing a pie that uses a purchased piecrust, simply tear out the paper label on the plastic cover (but do check it for a coupon good on a future purchase) and turn the cover upside down over the prepared pie. You now have a cover that protects your beautifully garnished pie from having anything fall on top of it. It makes the pie very portable when it's your turn to bring dessert to a get-together.

Did you know you can make your own **fruit-flavored yogurt?** Mix 1 tablespoon of any flavor of spreadable fruit spread with ¾ cup plain yogurt. It's every bit as tasty and much cheaper. You can also make your own **lemon yogurt** by combining 3 cups plain fat-free yogurt with 1 tub Crystal Light lemonade powder. Mix well, cover, and store in the refrigerator. I think you will be pleasantly surprised by the ease, cost, and flavor of this "made from scratch" calcium-rich treat. P.S.: You can make any flavor you like by using any of the Crystal Light mixes—Cranberry? Iced Tea? You decide.

Other Smart Substitutions

Many people have inquired about **substituting applesauce and artificial sweetener for butter and sugar**, but what if you aren't satisfied with the result? One woman wrote to me about a recipe for her grandmother's cookies that called for 1 cup of butter and 1½ cups of sugar. Well, any recipe that depends on as much butter and sugar as this one does is generally not a good candidate for "healthy exchanges." The original recipe needed a large quantity of fat to produce a crisp cookie just like Grandma made.

Applesauce can often be used instead of vegetable oil but generally doesn't work well as a replacement for butter, margarine, or lard. If a recipe calls for ½ cup of vegetable oil or less and your recipe is for a bar cookie, quick bread, muffin, or cake mix, you can try substituting an equal amount of unsweetened applesauce. If the recipe calls for more, try using ½ cup applesauce and the rest oil. You're cutting down the fat but shouldn't end up with a taste disaster! This "applesauce shortening" works great in many recipes, but so far I haven't been able to figure out a way to deep-fat fry with it!

Another rule for healthy substitution: Up to ½ cup sugar can be replaced by *an artificial sweetener that can withstand the heat of baking*, like pourable Sugar Twin or Sprinkle Sweet. If it requires more than ½ cup sugar, cut the amount needed by 75 percent and use ½ cup sugar substitute and sugar for the rest. Other options: Reduce the butter and sugar by 25 percent and see if the finished product still satisfies you in taste and appearance. Or, make the cookies just like Grandma did, realizing they are part of your family's holiday tradition. Enjoy a *moderate* serving of a couple of cookies once or twice during the season, and just forget about them the rest of the year.

Did you know that you can replace the fat in many quick breads, muffins, and shortcakes with **fat-free mayonnaise** or **fat-free sour cream?** This can work if the original recipe doesn't call for a lot of fat *and* sugar. If the recipe is truly fat and sugar dependent, such as traditional sugar cookies, cupcakes, or pastries, it won't work. Those recipes require the large amounts of sugar and fat to make love in the dark of the oven to produce a tender finished product. But if you have a favorite quick bread that doesn't call for a lot of sugar or fat, why don't you give one of these substitutes a try?

If you enjoy beverage mixes like those from Alba, here are my Healthy Exchanges versions:

For **chocolate-flavored,** use ⅓ cup nonfat dry milk powder and 2 tablespoons Nestlé Sugar-Free Chocolate Flavored Quik. Mix well and use as usual. Or, use ⅓ cup nonfat dry milk powder, 1 teaspoon unsweetened cocoa, and sugar substitute to equal 3 tablespoons sugar. Mix well and use as usual.

For **vanilla-flavored,** use ⅓ cup nonfat dry milk powder, sugar substitute to equal 2 tablespoons sugar, and add 1 teaspoon vanilla extract when adding liquid.

For **strawberry-flavored,** use ⅓ cup nonfat dry milk powder, sugar substitute to equal 2 tablespoons sugar, and add 1 teaspoon strawberry extract and 3–4 drops red food coloring when adding liquid.

Each of these makes one packet of drink mix. If you need to double the recipe, double everything but the extract. Use 1½ teaspoons of extract or it will be too strong. Use 1 cup cold water with one recipe mix to make a glass of flavored milk. If you want to make a shake, combine the mix, water, and 3–4 ice cubes in your blender, then process on BLEND till smooth.

A handy tip when making **healthy punch** for a party: Prepare a few extra cups of your chosen drink, freeze it in cubes in a couple of ice trays, then keep your punch from "watering down" by cooling it with punch cubes instead of ice cubes.

What should you do if you can't find the product listed in a Healthy Exchanges recipe? You can substitute in some cases—use Lemon JELL-O if you can't find Hawaiian Pineapple, for example. But if you're determined to track down the product you need, and your own store manager hasn't been able to order it for you, why not use one of the new online grocers and order exactly what you need, no matter where you live. Try **http://www.netgrocer.com.**

Not all low-fat cooking products are interchangeable, as one of my readers recently discovered when she tried to cook pancakes on her griddle using I Can't Believe It's Not Butter! spray— and they stuck! This butter-flavored spray is wonderful for a quick squirt on air-popped popcorn or corn on the cob, and it's great for topping your pancakes once they're cooked. In fact, my tastebuds have to check twice because it tastes so much like real butter! (And this is high praise from someone who once thought butter was the most perfect food ever created.)

But I Can't Believe It's Not Butter! doesn't work well for sautéing or browning. After trying to fry an egg with it and cooking up a disaster, I knew this product had its limitations. So I decided to continue using Pam or Weight Watchers butter-flavored cooking spray whenever I'm browning anything in a skillet or on a griddle.

Many of my readers have reported difficulty finding a product I use in many recipes: JELL-O cook-and-serve puddings. I have three suggestions for those of you with this problem:

1. **Work with your grocery store manager to get this product into your store**, and then make sure you and everyone you know buys it by the bagful! Products that sell well are reordered and kept in stock, especially with today's computerized cash registers that record what's purchased. You may also want to write or call Kraft General Foods and ask for their help. They can be reached at (800) 431-1001 weekdays from 9 A.M. to 4 P.M. (EST).

2. **You can prepare a recipe that calls for cook-and-serve pudding by using instant pudding of the same flavor.** Yes, that's right, you **can** cook with the instant when making my recipes. The finished product won't be quite as wonderful, but still at least a 3 on a 4-star scale. You can never do the opposite—never use cook-and-serve in a recipe that calls for instant! One time at a cooking demonstration, I could not understand why my Blueberry Mountain Cheesecake never did set up. Then I spotted the box in the trash and noticed I'd picked the wrong type of pudding mix. Be careful—the boxes are both blue, but the instant has pudding on a silver spoon, and the cook-and-serve has a stream of milk running down the front into a bowl with a wooden spoon.

3. **You can make JO's Sugar-Free Vanilla Cook-and-Serve Pudding Mix instead of using JELL-O's.** Here's my recipe: 2 tablespoons cornstarch, ½ cup pourable Sugar

Twin or Sprinkle Sweet, ⅔ cup Carnation Nonfat Dry Milk Powder, 1½ cups water, 2 teaspoons vanilla extract, and 4 to 5 drops yellow food coloring. Combine all this in a medium saucepan and cook over medium heat, stirring constantly, until the mixture comes to a full boil and thickens. This is for basic cooked vanilla sugar-free pudding. For a chocolate version, the recipe is 2 tablespoons cornstarch, ¼ cup pourable Sugar Twin or Sprinkle Sweet, 2 tablespoons sugar-free chocolate-flavored Nestlé's Quik, 1½ cups water, and 1 teaspoon vanilla extract. Follow the same cooking instructions as for the vanilla.

If you're preparing this as part of a recipe that also calls for adding a package of gelatin, just stir that into the mix.

Adapting a favorite family cake recipe? Here's something to try: Replace an egg and oil in the original with ⅓ cup fat-free yogurt and ¼ cup fat-free mayonnaise. Blend these two ingredients with your liquids in a separate bowl, then add the yogurt mixture to the flour mixture and mix gently just to combine. (You don't want to overmix or you'll release the gluten in the batter and end up with a tough batter.)

Want a tasty coffee creamer without all the fat? You could use Carnation's Fat Free Coffee-mate, which is 10 calories per teaspoon, but if you drink several cups a day with several teaspoons each, that adds up quickly to nearly 100 calories a day! Why not try my version? It's not quite as creamy, but it *is* good. Simply combine ⅓ cup Carnation Nonfat Dry Milk Powder and ¼ cup pourable Sugar Twin. Cover and store in your cupboard or refrigerator. At 3 calories per teaspoon, you can enjoy three teaspoons for less than the calories of one teaspoon of the purchased variety.

Some Helpful Hints

Sugar-free puddings and gelatins are important to many of my recipes, but if you prefer to avoid sugar substitutes, you could still prepare the recipes with regular puddings or gelatins. The calories would be higher, but you would still be cooking low-fat.

When a recipe calls for **chopped nuts** (and you only have whole ones), who wants to dirty the food processor just for a couple of tablespoonsful? You could try to chop them using your cutting board, but be prepared for bits and pieces to fly all over the kitchen. I use "Grandma's food processor." I take the biggest nuts I can find, put them in a small glass bowl, and chop them into chunks just the right size using a metal biscuit cutter.

A quick hint about **reduced-fat peanut butter:** Don't store it in the refrigerator. Because the fat has been reduced, it won't spread as easily when it's cold. Keep it in your cupboard and a little will spread a lot further.

Crushing **graham crackers** for topping? A self-seal sandwich bag works great!

If you have a **leftover muffin** and are looking for something a little different for breakfast, you can make **a "breakfast sundae."** Crumble the muffin into a cereal bowl. Sprinkle a serving of fresh fruit over it and top with a couple of tablespoons of plain fat-free yogurt sweetened with sugar substitute and your choice of extract. The thought of it just might make you jump out of bed with a smile on your face. (Speaking of muffins, did you know that if you fill the unused muffin wells with water when baking muffins, you help ensure more even baking and protect the muffin pan at the same time?) Another muffin hint: Lightly spray the inside of paper baking cups with butter-flavored cooking spray before spooning the muffin batter into them. Then you won't end up with paper clinging to your fresh-baked muffins.

The secret of making **good meringues** without sugar is to use 1 tablespoon of Sprinkle Sweet or pourable Sugar Twin for every egg white, and a small amount of extract. Use ½ to 1 teaspoon for the batch. Almond, vanilla, and coconut are all good choices. Use the same amount of cream of tartar you usually do. Bake the meringue in the same old way. Even if you can't eat sugar, you can enjoy a healthy meringue pie when it's prepared *The Healthy Exchanges Way*. (Remember that egg whites whip up best at room temperature.)

Try **storing your Bisquick Reduced Fat Baking Mix** in the freezer. It won't freeze, and it *will* stay fresh much longer. (It works for coffee, doesn't it?)

If you've ever wondered about **changing ingredients** in one of my recipes, the answer is that some things can be changed to suit your family's tastes, but others should not be tampered with. **Don't change**: the amount of flour, bread crumbs, reduced-fat baking mix, baking soda, baking powder, or liquid or dry milk powder. And if I include a small amount of salt, it's necessary for the recipe to turn out correctly. **What you can change:** an extract flavor (if you don't like coconut, choose vanilla or almond instead); a spreadable fruit flavor; the type of fruit in a pie filling (but be careful about substituting fresh for frozen and vice versa—sometimes it works, but it may not); the flavor of pudding or gelatin. As long as package sizes and amounts are the same, go for it. It will never hurt my feelings if you change a recipe, so please your family—don't worry about me!

Because I always say that "good enough" isn't good enough for me anymore, here's a way to make your cup of **fat-free and sugar-free hot cocoa** more special. After combining the hot chocolate mix and hot water, stir in ½ teaspoon vanilla extract and a light sprinkle of cinnamon. If you really want to feel decadent, add a tablespoon of Cool Whip Lite. Isn't life grand?

If you must limit your sugar intake, but you love the idea of sprinkling **powdered sugar** on dessert crepes or burritos, here's a pretty good substitute: Place 1 cup Sprinkle Sweet or pourable Sugar Twin and 1 teaspoon cornstarch in a blender container, then cover and process on HIGH until the mixture resembles powdered sugar in texture, about 45 to 60 seconds. Store in an airtight container and use whenever you want a dusting of "powdered sugar" on any dessert.

Want my "almost instant" pies to set up even more quickly? Do as one of my readers does: freeze your Keebler piecrusts. Then, when you stir up one of my pies and pour the filling into the frozen crust, it sets up within seconds.

Some of my "island-inspired" recipes call for **rum or brandy extracts** which provide the "essence" of liquor without the real thing. I'm a teetotaler by choice, so I choose not to include real liquor in any of my recipes. They're cheaper than liquor and you won't feel the need to shoo your kids away from the goodies. If you prefer not to use liquor extracts in your cooking, you can always substitute vanilla extract.

Some Healthy Cooking Challenges and How I Solved 'Em

When you stir up one of my pie fillings, do you ever have a problem with **lumps?** Here's an easy solution for all of you "careful" cooks out there. Lumps occur when the pudding starts to set up before you can get the dry milk powder incorporated into the mixture. I always advise you to dump, pour, and stir fast with that wire whisk, letting no more than 30 seconds elapse from beginning to end.

But if you are still having problems, you can always combine the dry milk powder and the water in a separate bowl before adding the pudding mix and whisking quickly. Why don't I suggest this right from the beginning? Because that would mean an extra dish to wash every time—and you know I hate to wash dishes!

With a little practice and a light touch, you should soon get the hang of my original method. But now you've got an alternative way to lose those lumps!

I love the chemistry of foods, and so I've gotten great pleasure from analyzing what makes fat-free products tick. By dissecting these "miracle" products, I've learned how to make them work best. They require different handling than the high-fat products we're used to, but if treated properly, these slimmed-down versions can produce delicious results!

Fat-free sour cream: This product is wonderful on a hot baked potato, but have you noticed that it tends to be much gummier than regular sour cream? If you want to use it in a stroganoff dish or baked product, you must stir a tablespoon or two of skim milk into the fat-free sour cream before adding it to other ingredients.

Cool Whip Free: When the fat went out of the formula, air was stirred in to fill the void. So, if you stir it too vigorously, you release the air and *decrease* the volume. Handle it with kid gloves— gently. Since the manufacturer forgot to ask for my input, I'll share with you how to make it taste almost the same as it used to. Let the container thaw in the refrigerator, then ever so gently stir in 1 teaspoon vanilla extract. Now, put the lid back on and enjoy it a tablespoon at a time, the same way you did Cool Whip Lite.

Fat-free cream cheese: When the fat was removed from this product, water replaced it. So don't ever use an electric mixer on the fat-free version, or you risk releasing the water and having your finished product look more like dip than cheesecake! Stirring it gently with a sturdy spoon in a glass bowl with a handle will soften it just as much as it needs to be. And don't be alarmed if the cream cheese gets caught in your wire whisk when you start combining the pudding mix and other ingredients. Just keep knocking it back down into the bowl by hitting the whisk against the rim of the bowl, and as you continue blending, it will soften even more and drop off the whisk. When it's time to pour the filling into your crust, your whisk shouldn't have anything much clinging to it.

Reduced-fat margarine: Again, the fat was replaced by water. If you try to use the reduced-fat kind in your cookie recipe spoon for spoon, you will end up with a cakelike cookie instead of the crisp kind most of us enjoy. You have to take into consideration that some water will be released as the product bakes. Use less liquid than the recipe calls for (when re-creating family recipes *only*—I've figured that into Healthy Exchanges recipes). And never, never, never use fat-*free* margarine and expect anyone to ask for seconds!

Homemade or Store-Bought?

I've been asked which is better for you: homemade from scratch, or purchased foods. My answer is *both!* Each has a place in a healthy lifestyle, and what that place is has everything to do with you.

Take **piecrusts,** for instance. If you love spending your spare time in the kitchen preparing foods, and you're using low-fat, low-sugar, and reasonably low-sodium ingredients, go for it! But if, like so many people, your time is limited and you've learned to read labels, you could be better off using purchased foods.

I know that when I prepare a pie (and I experiment with a couple of pies each week, because this is Cliff's favorite dessert), I use a purchased crust. Why? Mainly because I can't make a good-tasting piecrust that is lower in fat than the brands I use. Also, purchased piecrusts fit my rule of "If it takes longer to fix than to eat, forget it!"

I've checked the nutrient information for the purchased

piecrusts against recipes for traditional and "diet" piecrusts, using my computer software program. The purchased crust calculated lower in both fat and calories! I have tried some low-fat and low-sugar recipes, but they just didn't spark my tastebuds, or were so complicated you needed an engineering degree just to get the crust in the pie plate.

I'm very happy with the purchased piecrusts in my recipes, because the finished product rarely, if ever, has more than 30 percent of total calories coming from fats. I also believe that we have to prepare foods our families and friends will eat with us on a regular basis and not feel deprived, or we've wasted time, energy, and money.

I could use a purchased "lite" **pie filling,** but instead I make my own. Here I can save both fat and sugar, and still make the filling almost as fast as opening a can. The bottom line: Know what you have to spend when it comes to both time and fat/sugar calories, then make the best decision you can for you and your family. And don't go without an occasional piece of pie because you think it isn't *necessary.* A delicious pie prepared in a healthy way is one of the simple pleasures of life. It's a little thing, but it can make all the difference between just getting by with the bare minimum and living a full and healthy lifestyle.

I'm sure you'll add to this list of cooking tips as you begin preparing Healthy Exchanges recipes and discover how easy it can be to adapt your own favorite recipes using these ideas and your own common sense.

A Peek into My Pantry and My Favorite Brands

Everyone asks me what foods I keep on hand and what brands I use. There are lots of good products on the grocery shelves today—many more than we dreamed about even a year or two ago. And I can't wait to see what's out there twelve months from now. The following are my staples and, where appropriate, my favorites *at this time*. I feel these products are healthier, tastier, easy to get— and deliver the most flavor for the least amount of fat, sugar, or calories. If you find others you like as well *or better,* please use them. This is only a guide to make your grocery shopping and cooking easier.

> Plain fat-free yogurt (*Dannon—Yoplait no longer makes it*)
> Nonfat dry milk powder (*Carnation*)
> Evaporated skim milk (*Carnation*)
> Skim milk
> Fat-free cottage cheese
> Fat-free cream cheese (*Philadelphia*)
> Fat-free mayonnaise (*Kraft*)
> Fat-free salad dressings (*Kraft*)
> No-fat sour cream (*Land O Lakes*)
> Reduced-calorie margarine (*Weight Watchers, Promise, or Smart Beat*)
> Cooking spray
>> Olive oil–flavored (*Pam*)
>> Butter-flavored for sautéing (*Pam or Weight Watchers*)

Butter-flavored for spritzing *after* cooking (*I Can't Believe It's Not Butter!*)

Cooking oil (*Puritan Canola Oil*)

Reduced-calorie whipped topping (*Cool Whip Lite or Cool Whip Free*)

Sugar substitute
   if no heating is involved (*Equal*)
   if heating is required
      white (*pourable Sugar Twin*)
      brown (*Brown Sugar Twin*)

Sugar-free gelatin and pudding mixes (*JELL-O*)

Baking mix (*Bisquick Reduced Fat*)

Pancake mix (*Aunt Jemima Reduced Calorie*)

Reduced-calorie pancake syrup (*Cary's or Log Cabin*)

Parmesan cheese (*Kraft fat-free*)

Reduced-fat cheeses (shredded and sliced) (*Kraft Reduced Fat*)

Shredded frozen potatoes (*Mr. Dell's or Ore-Ida*)

Spreadable fruit spread (*Smucker's, Welch's or Knott's Berry Farm*)

Peanut butter (*Peter Pan reduced-fat, Jif reduced-fat, or Skippy reduced-fat*)

Chicken broth (*Healthy Request*)

Beef broth (*Swanson*)

Tomato sauce (*Hunt's*)

Canned soups (*Healthy Request*)

Tomato juice (*Healthy Request*)

Ketchup (*Heinz Light Harvest or Healthy Choice*)

Purchased piecrust
   unbaked (*Pillsbury—from dairy case*)
   graham cracker, shortbread, or chocolate-flavored (*Keebler*)

Crescent rolls (*Pillsbury Reduced Fat*)

Pastrami and corned beef (*Carl Buddig Lean*)

Luncheon meats (*Healthy Choice or Oscar Mayer*)

Ham (*Dubuque 97% fat-free or Healthy Choice*)

Frankfurters and kielbasa sausage (*Healthy Choice*)

Canned white chicken, packed in water (*Chicken of the Sea*)

Canned tuna, packed in water (*Starkist or Chicken of the Sea*)

90 to 97 percent lean ground turkey and beef

Soda crackers (*Nabisco Fat-Free*)
Reduced-calorie bread—40 calories per slice or less
Hamburger buns—80 calories each
Rice—instant, regular, and wild
Instant potato flakes
Noodles, spaghetti, and macaroni
Salsa (*Chi-Chi's or Pace Mild Chunky*)
Pickle relish—dill, sweet, and hot dog
Mustard—Dijon, prepared, and spicy
Unsweetened apple and orange juice
Unsweetened applesauce
Fruit—fresh, frozen (no sugar added), or canned in juice
Vegetables—fresh, frozen, or canned
Spices—JO's Spices or any national brand
Lemon and lime juice (in small plastic fruit-shaped bottles found in the produce section)
Instant fruit beverage mixes (*Crystal Light*)
Sugar-free chocolate beverage mixes—cold and hot (*Nestlé Quik*)
Sugar-free and fat-free ice cream—*Wells' Blue Bunny Health Beat*

The items on my shopping list are everyday foods found in just about any grocery store in America. But all are as low in fat, sugar, calories, and sodium as I can find—and still taste good! I can make any recipe in my cookbooks and newsletters as long as I have my cupboards and refrigerator stocked with these items. Whenever I use the last of any one item, I just make sure I pick up another supply the next time I'm at the store.

If your grocer does not stock these items, why not ask if they can be ordered on a trial basis? If the store agrees to do so, be sure to tell your friends to stop by, so that sales are good enough to warrant restocking the new products. Competition for shelf space is fierce, so only products that sell well stay around.

How to Read a Healthy Exchanges Recipe

The Healthy Exchanges Nutritional Analysis

Before using these recipes, you may wish to consult your physician or health-care provider to be sure they are appropriate for you. The information in this book is not intended to take the place of any medical advice. It reflects my experiences, studies, research, and opinions regarding healthy eating.

Each recipe includes nutritional information calculated in three ways:

> Healthy Exchanges Weight Loss Choices™ or Exchanges
> Calories; Fat, Protein, Carbohydrates, and Fiber in grams;
> Sodium and Calcium in milligrams
> Diabetic Exchanges

In every Healthy Exchanges recipe, the diabetic exchanges have been calculated by a registered dietitian. All the other calculations were done by computer, using the Food Processor II software. When the ingredient listing gives more than one choice, the first ingredient listed is the one used in the recipe analysis. Due to inevitable variations in the ingredients you choose to use, the nutritional values should be considered approximate.

The annotation "(limited)" following Protein counts in some recipes indicates that consumption of whole eggs should be limited to four per week.

Please note the following symbols:

☆ This star means read the recipe's directions carefully for special instructions about **division** of ingredients.

❄ This symbol indicates **FREEZES WELL.**

The Recipes

Soups

Savory Tomato Soup

It was always the perfect definition of comfort food when you were just a kid, but now you're all grown-up, and so is this flavorful version of an old-fashioned favorite. Smooth and creamy, it's oh-so-satisfying for a Sunday supper or anyday lunch!

⊙   Serves 4 (1 full cup)

> 1 (10¾-ounce) can Healthy Request Tomato Soup
> 1¾ cups (one 15-ounce can) Hunt's Tomato Sauce
> 1 teaspoon dried minced garlic
> 1 teaspoon dried onion flakes
> 1 tablespoon dried basil
> 2 teaspoons dried parsley flakes
> 1⅓ cups skim milk
> ¼ cup (¾ ounce) grated Kraft fat-free Parmesan cheese

In a large saucepan, combine tomato soup, tomato sauce, garlic, onion flakes, basil, and parsley flakes. Mix well to combine. Add skim milk and Parmesan cheese. Mix well to combine. Lower heat and simmer for 10 minutes or until mixture is heated through, stirring occasionally.

Each serving equals:

HE: 1¾ Vegetable • ⅓ Skim Milk • ¼ Protein • ½ Slider • 5 Optional Calories

76 Calories • 0 gm Fat • 4 gm Protein • 15 gm Carbohydrate • 855 mg Sodium • 105 mg Calcium • 1 gm Fiber

DIABETIC: 2 Vegetable • ½ Starch

Chunky Tomato Soup

Hungry men—and women—step right up! This soup is hearty and brimful of tasty goodness. The blend of flavors will awaken taste-buds you didn't know you had! ☻ Serves 4 (1¼ cups)

½ cup chopped onion
1¾ cups (one 14½-ounce can) Swanson Beef Broth
1 (10¾-ounce) can Healthy Request Tomato Soup
1 teaspoon Italian seasoning
½ teaspoon Worcestershire sauce
1½ cups peeled and chopped fresh tomatoes
1½ cups chopped unpeeled zucchini

In a medium saucepan sprayed with olive oil–flavored cooking spray, sauté onion for 5 minutes or just until tender. Add beef broth, tomato soup, Italian seasoning, and Worcestershire sauce. Mix well to combine. Stir in tomatoes and zucchini. Bring mixture to a boil. Lower heat and simmer for 5 to 6 minutes or until vegetables are just tender, stirring often.

Each serving equals:

HE: 1¾ Vegetable • ½ Slider • 14 Optional Calories

94 Calories • 2 gm Fat • 3 gm Protein •
16 gm Carbohydrate • 604 mg Sodium •
23 mg Calcium • 2 gm Fiber

DIABETIC: 1 Starch/Carbohydrate or 2 Vegetable •
½ Starch/Carbohydrate

Grande Cream of Tomato Soup

Here's a sweet and tangy, rich and luscious way to prepare a truly festive tomato soup. You get a great calcium boost in every bowl, and if you're like Cliff (Mr. Spice-is-nice!) you can increase the chili seasoning *carefully* to make this even hotter!

☻ Serves 2 (1½ cups)

> 1 cup skim milk
> 1¾ cups (one 14½-ounce can) stewed tomatoes, undrained
> 1½ tablespoons all-purpose flour
> 1 tablespoon pourable Sugar Twin
> 1½ teaspoons chili seasoning
> ⅛ teaspoon black pepper

In a medium saucepan, cook skim milk until hot, but not boiling, stirring often. Meanwhile, in a blender container, combine undrained stewed tomatoes, flour, Sugar Twin, chili seasoning, and black pepper. Cover and process on BLEND for 10 seconds. Add hot milk. Re-cover and continue processing on BLEND for 15 seconds. Pour mixture back into saucepan. Continue cooking for 3 to 4 minutes or until mixture is heated through, stirring constantly.

Each serving equals:

HE: 1¾ Vegetable • ½ Skim Milk • ¼ Bread •
3 Optional Calories

160 Calories • 0 gm Fat • 11 gm Protein •
29 gm Carbohydrate • 658 mg Sodium •
303 mg Calcium • 2 gm Fiber

DIABETIC: 2 Vegetable • ½ Skim Milk

Jamaican Carrot Soup

You will quickly feel warmed by the Caribbean sun when you spoon up this island-inspired dish that brings the tropics close to home! It's amazing how just a dab of peanut butter gives this soup its delightful flavor—and how a bit of Tabasco turns up the volume!

○ Serves 2 (¾ cup)

> ½ cup chopped onion
> 2 cups (one 16-ounce can) Healthy Request Chicken Broth
> ½ teaspoon dried minced garlic
> 1½ cups grated carrots
> 1 tablespoon Peter Pan reduced-fat chunky peanut butter
> 1 to 2 drops Tabasco sauce

In a medium saucepan sprayed with butter-flavored cooking spray, sauté onion about 5 minutes or until tender. Add chicken broth, garlic, and carrots. Mix well to combine. Lower heat, cover, and simmer for 15 minutes, or until carrots are tender. Pour mixture into a blender container. Add peanut butter and Tabasco sauce. Cover and process on BLEND for about 30 to 45 seconds or until mixture is smooth. Serve at once.

Each serving equals:

> HE: 2 Vegetable • ½ Fat • ½ Protein •
> 16 Optional Calories
> _____
> 107 Calories • 3 gm Fat • 6 gm Protein •
> 14 gm Carbohydrate • 538 mg Sodium •
> 24 mg Calcium • 3 gm Fiber
> _____
> DIABETIC: 1½ Vegetable • ½ Starch/Carbohydrate •
> ½ Fat • or 1 Starch/Carbohydrate • ½ Fat

Potato and Carrot Soup

Potato soup was always one of my favorite comfort dishes when I was growing up, and I try to include at least one potato-based soup in all of my recipe collections. This one is thick and soothing, a wonderful complement to a sandwich on a cold winter day.

🌑 Serves 4 (1½ cups)

½ cup finely chopped onion
3 cups (15 ounces) diced raw potatoes
1½ cups water
1 cup shredded carrots
½ teaspoon lemon pepper
3 tablespoons all-purpose flour
2 cups skim milk
1 teaspoon dried parsley flakes
¼ cup Hormel Bacon Bits

In a large saucepan sprayed with butter-flavored cooking spray, sauté onion for 5 minutes or just until tender. Add potatoes and water. Mix well to combine. Bring mixture to a boil. Lower heat, cover, and simmer for 15 minutes. Stir in carrots and lemon pepper. In a covered jar, combine flour, skim milk, and parsley flakes. Shake well to blend. Stir milk mixture into potato mixture. Continue simmering until mixture slightly thickens, stirring often. Just before serving, stir in bacon bits.

Each serving equals:

HE: 1 Bread • ¾ Vegetable • ½ Skim Milk • ¼ Slider • 5 Optional Calories

---

178 Calories • 2 gm Fat • 10 gm Protein • 30 gm Carbohydrate • 328 mg Sodium • 170 mg Calcium • 2 gm Fiber

---

DIABETIC: 1½ Starch • ½ Vegetable • ½ Skim Milk

Corn-Celery Chowder

Cooking in the microwave makes sense for lots of reasons, but one of the best is that you can cook and serve your recipe in the same bowl! This fast and fabulous chowder sparkles with delectable corn flavor, and it's a great choice on nights when you've got only minutes to whip up dinner.　　◐　Serves 4 (1¼ cups)

¾ cup finely chopped celery

¼ cup finely chopped onion

1 cup + 2 tablespoons water ☆

1 cup (one 8-ounce can) cream-style corn

1 cup (one 8-ounce can) whole-kernel corn, undrained

⅔ cup Carnation Nonfat Dry Milk Powder

1 (10¾-ounce) can Healthy Request Cream of Celery Soup

1 teaspoon dried parsley flakes

⅛ teaspoon black pepper

2 tablespoons Hormel Bacon Bits

In an 8-cup glass measuring bowl, combine celery, onion, and 2 tablespoons water. Cover and microwave on HIGH (100% power) for 5 minutes or until celery is tender. Stir in cream-style corn and undrained whole-kernel corn. In a small bowl, combine remaining 1 cup water and dry milk powder. Stir in celery soup, parsley flakes, and black pepper. Add milk mixture to celery mixture. Mix well to combine. Re-cover and continue to microwave on HIGH for 5 minutes. Stir in bacon bits. Let set for 1 to 2 minutes before serving.

Each serving equals:

HE: 1 Bread • ½ Skim Milk • ½ Vegetable •
½ Slider • 14 Optional Calories

---

199 Calories • 3 gm Fat • 8 gm Protein •
35 gm Carbohydrate • 851 mg Sodium •
205 mg Calcium • 2 gm Fiber

DIABETIC: 1½ Starch • ½ Skim Milk

Fireside Corn Chowder

Back when President Roosevelt spoke to the nation in his fireside chats, whole families gathered around the radio to hear his words of comfort and inspiration. I like to think this is the kind of soup they might have enjoyed while listening to him. It's quick, it's filling, it's inexpensive to prepare. Why, it could be your patriotic duty to serve it soon!   ☻   Serves 2 (1¼ cups)

> ½ cup finely chopped onion
> Scant 1 cup (4 ounces) diced cooked potatoes
> 1 cup skim milk
> 1 cup (one 8-ounce can) cream-style corn
> 2 tablespoons Hormel Bacon Bits
> 1 teaspoon dried parsley flakes

In a medium saucepan sprayed with butter-flavored cooking spray, sauté onion for 5 minutes or until tender. Add potatoes, skim milk, and corn. Mix well to combine. Stir in bacon bits and parsley flakes. Bring mixture to a boil. Lower heat and simmer for 5 minutes or until heated through, stirring occasionally.

Each serving equals:

HE: 1½ Bread • ½ Skim Milk • ¼ Vegetable • ¼ Slider • 5 Optional Calories

222 Calories • 2 gm Fat • 12 gm Protein • 39 gm Carbohydrate • 530 mg Sodium • 218 mg Calcium • 3 gm Fiber

DIABETIC: 2 Starch • ½ Skim Milk • ½ Fat

Easy Clam Chowder

A lot of people only enjoy clam chowder when they are traveling to parts of the country where it's usually on the menu, especially New England. But why should you deny yourself the pleasure of this tasty soup the rest of the year? Here's a version that will make it a regular on your table!   ☻   Serves 4 (1 cup)

½ cup finely chopped onion
2 cups (one 16-ounce can) cream-style corn
1 (6.5-ounce drained weight) can minced clams, undrained
1 teaspoon seafood seasoning
⅔ cup Carnation Nonfat Dry Milk Powder
1¼ cups water

In a medium saucepan sprayed with butter-flavored cooking spray, sauté onion for 5 minutes or until tender. Stir in corn, undrained clams, and seafood seasoning. In a small bowl, combine dry milk powder and water. Add milk mixture to clam mixture. Mix well to combine. Lower heat and simmer for 5 minutes, stirring occasionally.

Each serving equals:

HE: 1⅔ Protein • 1 Bread • ½ Skim Milk • ¼ Vegetable

---

213 Calories • 1 gm Fat • 18 gm Protein • 33 gm Carbohydrate • 479 mg Sodium • 188 mg Calcium • 2 gm Fiber

---

DIABETIC: 1½ Meat • 1½ Starch • ½ Skim Milk

Turkey-Rice Soup

When I was creating this recipe, I half-remembered a children's rhyme that said something about oh dear, how nice, to eat chicken soup with rice. Yes, it certainly is—and so is this cozy combo of turkey with that beloved grain! This is a wonderful dish to stir up when you've got Thanksgiving leftovers, but turkey isn't just for holidays anymore.   ❂   Serves 4 (1½ cups)

> 1 cup water
> 1½ cups (8 ounces) diced cooked turkey breast
> 4 cups (two 16-ounce cans) Healthy Request Chicken Broth
> 1 cup shredded carrots
> 1 cup finely chopped celery
> 1 tablespoon dried parsley flakes
> ⅛ teaspoon black pepper
> 1 cup (3 ounces) uncooked instant Minute Rice

In a large saucepan, combine water, turkey, and chicken broth. Add carrots, celery, parsley flakes, and black pepper. Mix well to combine. Bring mixture to a boil. Stir in uncooked rice. Lower heat, cover, and simmer for 20 to 25 minutes, stirring occasionally.

HINT: If you don't have leftovers, purchase a chunk of cooked turkey breast from your local deli.

Each serving equals:

HE: 2 Protein • 1 Vegetable • ¾ Bread •
16 Optional Calories

174 Calories • 2 gm Fat • 22 gm Protein •
17 gm Carbohydrate • 552 mg Sodium •
33 mg Calcium • 1 gm Fiber

DIABETIC: 2 Meat • 1 Vegetable • 1 Starch

Turkey Soup and Dumplings Duo

Two can be better than one when two people are happier married than they are on their own. (Just ask Cliff and me!) The same is true of turkey soup and dumplings. They're plenty tasty on their own, but together theirs is a marriage made in cookbook heaven!

◐ Serves 4 (1½ cups)

2 cups (one 16-ounce can) Healthy Request Chicken Broth	2 cups (10 ounces) diced cooked turkey breast
2 cups water	¾ cup Bisquick Reduced Fat Baking Mix
1 cup sliced carrots	1 teaspoon dried parsley flakes
1 cup sliced celery	½ cup skim milk
1 teaspoon dried onion flakes	

In an 8-cup glass measuring bowl, combine chicken broth, water, carrots, celery, onion flakes, and turkey. Cover and microwave on HIGH (100% power) for 6 to 8 minutes or until vegetables are tender. In a medium bowl, combine baking mix, parsley flakes, and skim milk. Drop by spoonfuls into hot mixture to form 8 dumplings. Re-cover and continue to microwave on HIGH for 4 to 5 minutes or until dumplings are light and springy to touch, and no longer doughy. Let set for 2 minutes before serving.

HINT: If you don't have leftovers, purchase a chunk of cooked turkey breast from your local deli.

Each serving equals:

HE: 2½ Protein • 1 Bread • 1 Vegetable • 19 Optional Calories

178 Calories • 2 gm Fat • 17 gm Protein • 23 gm Carbohydrate • 825 mg Sodium • 78 mg Calcium • 2 gm Fiber

DIABETIC: 2½ Meat • 1 Starch • 1 Vegetable

Grandma's Soup Pot

I love this recipe, and so did my family when I tried it out on them. I said, "Grandma's refrigerator was filled with little bits of this and that, so I tossed them all into my soup pot!" Here's the happy result—a rich and satisfying melange of healthy foods, all joined in a happy family hug!   ❂   Serves 8 (1½ cups)

16 ounces ground 90% lean
   turkey or beef
1 cup diced onion
1¾ cups (one 15-ounce can)
   Swanson Beef Broth
4½ cups water
1¾ cups (one 15-ounce can)
   Hunt's Tomato Sauce
1 cup sliced fresh carrots
1 cup diced celery

1½ cups shredded cabbage
1 cup (5 ounces) diced raw
   potatoes
⅔ cup (2 ounces) uncooked
   instant Minute Rice
⅛ teaspoon black pepper
2 teaspoons dried parsley
   flakes
½ cup frozen peas

In a large saucepan sprayed with butter-flavored cooking spray, brown meat and onion. Stir in beef broth, water, and tomato sauce. Add carrots, celery, cabbage, potatoes, and uncooked rice. Mix well to combine. Bring mixture to a boil. Stir in black pepper and parsley flakes. Lower heat, cover, and simmer for 30 minutes, stirring occasionally. Add peas. Mix well to combine. Continue simmering for 5 minutes, stirring occasionally.

Each serving equals:

HE: 2 Vegetable • 1½ Protein • ½ Bread •
4 Optional Calories

157 Calories • 5 gm Fat • 13 gm Protein •
15 gm Carbohydrate • 608 mg Sodium •
27 mg Calcium • 3 gm Fiber

DIABETIC: 2 Vegetable • 1½ Meat • ½ Starch

Country Vegetable Soup

It turns up on the menu of every cozy country inn across America—a flavorful, old-fashioned veggie soup that warms you inside and out. Here's my easy-to-fix version that can simmer for hours without being watched!   ☻   Serves 6 (1½ cups)

16 ounces ground 90% lean turkey or beef
¾ cup chopped onion
1¾ cups (one 14½-ounce can) stewed tomatoes, undrained
1 cup (one 8-ounce can) Hunt's Tomato Sauce
1 cup water
1¾ cups (one 14½-ounce can) Swanson Beef Broth
1 tablespoon Brown Sugar Twin
2 cups frozen cut carrots
1¾ cups frozen cut green beans
1 cup frozen peas
2 cups (10 ounces) diced raw potatoes
1 teaspoon dried parsley flakes

In a large saucepan sprayed with butter-flavored cooking spray, brown meat and onion. Spoon mixture into a slow cooker container. Add undrained tomatoes, tomato sauce, water, beef broth, and Brown Sugar Twin. Mix well to combine. Stir in carrots, green beans, peas, potatoes, and parsley flakes. Cover and cook on LOW for 6 to 8 hours. Mix well just before serving.

Each serving equals:

HE: 2½ Vegetable • 2 Protein • ¾ Bread •
7 Optional Calories

215 Calories • 7 gm Fat • 17 gm Protein •
21 gm Carbohydrate • 807 mg Sodium •
66 mg Calcium • 4 gm Fiber

DIABETIC: 2½ Vegetable • 2 Meat • 1 Starch

Lone Star Corn Chili

I bet one of these years the Iowa State Fair will decide to put on a corn chili cook-off! After all, chili is a family favorite in every part of the country, and corn is our unofficial state vegetable. (Maybe I'll call the governor and suggest it. . . .) I call this Lone Star in honor of Texas, where Cliff and I have eaten many great cups of chili.

◎ Serves 4 (1½ cups)

> 8 ounces ground 90% lean turkey or beef
> ½ cup chopped onion
> ½ cup chopped green bell pepper
> 2 cups (one 16-ounce can) tomatoes, coarsely
>   chopped and undrained
> 2 cups Healthy Request tomato juice or any reduced-sodium
>   tomato juice
> 1½ cups frozen whole-kernel corn
> 1½ teaspoons chili seasoning
> ⅓ cup (1½ ounces) shredded Kraft reduced-fat Cheddar cheese

In a large saucepan sprayed with olive oil–flavored cooking spray, brown meat, onion, and green pepper. Stir in undrained tomatoes and tomato juice. Add corn and chili seasoning. Mix well to combine. Bring mixture to a boil. Lower heat and simmer for 10 minutes, stirring occasionally. When serving, sprinkle 1½ table-spoons Cheddar cheese over top of each bowl.

Each serving equals:

> HE: 2½ Vegetable • 2 Protein • ¾ Bread
>
> ---
>
> 223 Calories • 7 gm Fat • 16 gm Protein •
> 24 gm Carbohydrate • 354 mg Sodium •
> 119 mg Calcium • 4 gm Fiber
>
> ---
>
> DIABETIC: 2 Vegetable • 2 Meat • 1 Starch

End-of-Summer Chili

Wouldn't this be a great dish to serve at a Labor Day cookout, the last big party before the kids head back to school? This tasty version will please everyone but my son Tommy, who still skips out when kidney beans are on the menu. (I warned Angie before she married him, but she told me it wasn't a deal-breaker!)

☻ Serves 4 (1½ cups)

> 8 ounces ground 90% lean turkey or beef
> ½ cup chopped green bell pepper
> ½ cup chopped onion
> 10 ounces (one 16-ounce can) red kidney beans,
>   rinsed and drained
> 1 cup (one 8-ounce can) Hunt's Tomato Sauce
> 2 cups peeled and chopped fresh tomatoes
> 2 cups water
> 2 tablespoons chili seasoning

In a large saucepan sprayed with olive oil–flavored cooking spray, brown meat, green pepper, and onion. Stir in kidney beans. Add tomato sauce, tomatoes, water, and chili seasoning. Mix well to combine. Bring mixture to a boil. Lower heat and simmer for 15 to 20 minutes, stirring occasionally.

Each serving equals:

HE: 2¾ Protein • 2½ Vegetable

189 Calories • 5 gm Fat • 15 gm Protein • 21 gm Carbohydrate • 464 mg Sodium • 27 mg Calcium • 7 gm Fiber

DIABETIC: 2 Vegetable • 1 Starch • ½ Meat

Steakhouse Soup

Here's a sensational soup for those nights when everyone tells you, "I'm really, *really* hungry!" It's just jam-packed with meat and veggies, a true meal-in-a-bowl that lets your tummy know you care! And because it's prepared in the microwave, all those flavors join hands in a hurry. ☻ Serves 6 (1 cup)

1½ cups frozen sliced carrots, thawed
1½ cups frozen cut green beans, thawed
1¾ cups (one 14½-ounce can) Swanson Beef Broth
1 full cup (6 ounces) finely diced cooked lean roast beef

¾ cup frozen peas, thawed
¾ cup frozen whole-kernel corn, thawed
Scant 1 cup (4 ounces) diced cooked potatoes
2 teaspoons dried onion flakes
1 teaspoon dried parsley flakes
1 (12-ounce) jar Heinz Fat Free Beef Gravy

In an 8-cup glass measuring bowl, combine carrots, green beans, and beef broth. Cover and microwave on HIGH (100% power) for 6 minutes, stirring after 3 minutes. Stir in roast beef, peas, corn, potatoes, onion flakes, parsley flakes, and beef gravy. Re-cover and continue to microwave on HIGH for 6 to 8 minutes, or until vegetables are tender. Let set for 5 minutes before serving.

HINTS: 1. Thaw frozen vegetables by placing in a colander and rinsing under hot water for one minute.
2. If you don't have leftovers, purchase a chunk of cooked roast beef from your local deli or use a 6-ounce package of Healthy Choice lean roast beef slices.

Each serving equals:

HE: 1 Protein • 1 Vegetable • ⅔ Bread • ¼ Slider • 11 Optional Calories

143 Calories • 2 gm Fat • 12 gm Protein • 17 gm Carbohydrate • 607 mg Sodium • 27 mg Calcium • 3 gm Fiber

DIABETIC: 1 Meat • 1 Vegetable • ½ Starch

French Quarter Onion Soup

It's a bistro classic, a rich, oniony broth topped with melted cheese, and traditionally served with a chunk of French bread. If you used to love ordering that high-calorie, high-fat version at restaurants, you'll be dazzled by how I've reinvented it for Healthy Exchanges. Stirring the cheese into the soup makes it so thick and tangy, another name for this dish might be "The Big Easy!"

○ Serves 4 (1½ cups)

> 3 cups thinly sliced onion
> 2 cups (one 16-ounce can) Healthy Request Chicken Broth
> 1 cup water
> 1 (10¾-ounce) can Healthy Request Cream of Celery Soup
> 1 teaspoon Worcestershire sauce
> 4 to 6 drops Tabasco sauce
> 1 full cup (6 ounces) diced Dubuque 97% fat-free ham or any
>   extra-lean ham
> 4 (¾-ounce) slices Kraft reduced-fat Swiss cheese, shredded

In a large saucepan sprayed with butter-flavored cooking spray, sauté onion for 8 to 10 minutes. Stir in chicken broth, water, celery soup, Worcestershire, and Tabasco sauce. Bring mixture to a boil. Add ham and Swiss cheese. Mix well to combine. Lower heat and simmer for 5 minutes, or until mixture is heated through and cheese melts, stirring occasionally.

Each serving equals:

HE: 2 Protein • 1½ Vegetable • ½ Slider •
5 Optional Calories

---

155 Calories • 3 gm Fat • 11 gm Protein •
21 gm Carbohydrate • 897 mg Sodium •
76 mg Calcium • 3 gm Fiber

DIABETIC: 2 Meat • 1½ Vegetable • ½ Starch

Great Northern Bean and Mac Soup

I get lots of questions asking what to do with all the different beans you find on your supermarket shelves, and coming up with tasty bean recipes is one of my favorite projects. (We're all trying to eat more beans and less meat to boost fiber!) This dish delivers lots of healthy protein, and the mixed-in macaroni makes you feel like a lucky kid!   ☻   Serves 4 (1½ cups)

> 2 cups (one 16-ounce can) Healthy Request
>   Chicken Broth
> 1 cup water
> 10 ounces (one 16-ounce can) great northern beans, rinsed
>   and drained
> ½ cup chopped onion
> 1 cup shredded carrots
> 1 cup finely chopped celery
> 1 full cup (6 ounces) diced Dubuque 97% fat-free ham
>   or any extra-lean ham
> ¼ cup (¾ ounce) grated Kraft fat-free
>   Parmesan cheese
> 1 teaspoon dried parsley flakes
> ⅛ teaspoon black pepper
> 1 cup hot cooked elbow macaroni, rinsed and drained

In a large saucepan, combine chicken broth, water, great northern beans, onion, carrots, and celery. Bring mixture to a boil. Stir in ham. Lower heat and simmer for 15 minutes or until vegetables are tender. Add Parmesan cheese, parsley flakes, black pepper, and macaroni. Mix well to combine. Continue simmering for 10 minutes, stirring occasionally.

HINT: ⅔ cup uncooked macaroni usually cooks to about 1 cup.

Each serving equals:

HE: 2½ Protein • 1¼ Vegetable • ½ Bread •
8 Optional Calories

226 Calories • 2 gm Fat • 17 gm Protein •
35 gm Carbohydrate • 708 mg Sodium •
76 mg Calcium • 6 gm Fiber

DIABETIC: 2 Meat • 1½ Starch • ½ Vegetable

Green Bean Soup with Ham

Here's a savory blend that's a real man-pleaser, and nowhere more than in my house, where the green bean is Vegetable Number One on Cliff's Top Ten List! This recipe is especially wonderful when the leaves start turning bright colors and that cold wind starts whipping across our Iowa plains. ● Serves 4 (1½ cups)

> 2 cups frozen cut green beans
> ½ cup chopped onion
> ½ cup frozen sliced carrots
> 2 cups (one 16-ounce can) Healthy Request Chicken Broth
> 1 cup water
> 1 full cup (6 ounces) diced Dubuque 97% fat-free ham or any
>   extra-lean ham
> 1 teaspoon dried parsley flakes
> ⅛ teaspoon black pepper
> ⅓ cup (1 ounce) uncooked instant Minute Rice

In a large saucepan, combine green beans, onion, carrots, chicken broth, and water. Bring mixture to a boil. Stir in ham, parsley flakes, and black pepper. Add uncooked rice. Mix well to combine. Lower heat, cover, and simmer for 15 to 20 minutes or until vegetables and rice are tender, stirring occasionally.

Each serving equals:

HE: 1½ Vegetable • 1 Protein • ¼ Bread •
8 Optional Calories

---

81 Calories • 1 gm Fat • 8 gm Protein •
10 gm Carbohydrate • 571 mg Sodium •
29 mg Calcium • 2 gm Fiber

DIABETIC: 2 Vegetable • 1 Meat

St. Pat's Potato Soup

Every ethnic group has contributed its favorite recipes to our American melting pot, and my own Irish ancestors were big fans of the potato. (It was such a staple of Irish diets, both in Ireland and over here!) I think you'll enjoy digging into cozy bowls of this yummy soup when you come home from cheering at the parade!

◑ Serves 4 (1⅓ cups)

> 2 cups (10 ounces) diced raw potatoes
> ½ cup chopped onion
> 2 cups chopped cabbage
> 1 cup hot water
> 3 cups skim milk
> 3 tablespoons all-purpose flour
> 1 (10¾-ounce) can Healthy Request Cream of Mushroom Soup
> 1 teaspoon dried parsley flakes
> 1 (2.5-ounce) package Carl Buddig 90% lean corned beef,
>   shredded

In a large saucepan, combine potatoes, onion, cabbage, and water. Cover and cook over medium heat for about 15 minutes or until potatoes are tender. In a covered jar, combine skim milk and flour. Shake well to blend. Pour milk mixture into undrained potato mixture. Add mushroom soup, parsley flakes, and corned beef. Mix well to combine. Lower heat and simmer for 10 minutes, or until mixture is heated through, stirring often.

Each serving equals:

HE: 1¼ Vegetable • ¾ Bread • ⅔ Protein •
½ Skim Milk • ½ Slider • 1 Optional Calorie

---

207 Calories • 3 gm Fat • 13 gm Protein •
32 gm Carbohydrate • 642 mg Sodium •
302 mg Calcium • 2 gm Fiber

DIABETIC: 1 Vegetable • 1 Starch • 1 Skim Milk •
½ Meat

Magic Minestrone

It almost seems supernatural how a handful of basic ingredients can be transformed into a spectacular soup that "eats like a meal!" Serving this with a salad and your favorite hearty bread makes a wonderfully satisfying meal. Presto! You're a star in your own kitchen!

○ Serves 4 (1¼ cups)

> 1 (2.5-ounce) package Carl Buddig lean pastrami, shredded
> ½ cup chopped onion
> 1 cup shredded carrots
> 1¾ cups (one 14½-ounce can) Swanson Beef Broth
> 1¾ cups (one 15-ounce can) Hunt's Tomato Sauce
> 1 teaspoon Italian seasoning
> 10 ounces (one 16-ounce can) great northern beans,
>   rinsed and drained
> ½ cup (1½ ounces) uncooked small shell macaroni
> 1½ cups chopped unpeeled zucchini
> ¼ cup (¾ ounce) grated Kraft fat-free Parmesan cheese

In a large saucepan sprayed with olive oil–flavored cooking spray, sauté pastrami, onion, and carrots until vegetables are just tender. Add beef broth, tomato sauce, and Italian seasoning. Mix well to combine. Bring mixture to a boil. Stir in great northern beans and uncooked macaroni. Lower heat, cover, and simmer for 10 minutes. Add zucchini. Mix well to combine. Re-cover and continue simmering for 5 minutes or until zucchini and macaroni are tender, stirring occasionally. When serving, sprinkle 1 tablespoon Parmesan cheese over top of each bowl.

Each serving equals:

HE: 3¼ Vegetable • 2 Protein • ½ Bread •
16 Optional Calories

234 Calories • 2 gm Fat • 15 gm Protein •
39 gm Carbohydrate • 941 mg Sodium •
69 mg Calcium • 8 gm Fiber

DIABETIC: 3 Vegetable • ½ Meat • ½ Starch

Savory Salads

Island Cabbage and Celery Salad

There's something so satisfying about the crunch of a savory salad, especially this one that doubles the pleasure with both celery and cabbage! You'll notice that I love to "doctor up" fat-free salad dressings to make them just a little bit more interesting and tasty than straight from the bottle.   ☻   Serves 4 (¾ cup)

2 cups shredded cabbage
1 cup chopped celery
⅓ cup Kraft Fat Free Thousand Island Dressing
2 tablespoons Kraft fat-free mayonnaise
1 teaspoon dried onion flakes
1 teaspoon dried parsley flakes
⅛ teaspoon black pepper

In a medium bowl, combine cabbage and celery. In a small bowl, combine Thousand Island dressing, mayonnaise, onion flakes, parsley flakes, and black pepper. Add dressing mixture to cabbage mixture. Mix gently to combine. Cover and refrigerate for at least 30 minutes. Gently stir again just before serving.

Each serving equals:

HE: 1½ Vegetable • ¼ Slider • 18 Optional Calories

44 Calories • 0 gm Fat • 0 gm Protein •
11 gm Carbohydrate • 275 mg Sodium •
31 mg Calcium • 1 gm Fiber

DIABETIC: 2 Vegetable

Turn-of-the-Century Slaw

Coleslaw is one of those great American classics that can be incredibly high-fat and unhealthy, or with a little Healthy Exchanges magic, amazingly tasty and good for you! Even if your old standby is your great-aunt's secret recipe, give this one a try and see if it delivers the flavor you love!   ❤   Serves 6 (¾ cup)

> ⅔ cup Carnation Nonfat Dry Milk Powder
> ½ cup water
> 1 tablespoon + 1 teaspoon white vinegar ☆
> ½ cup Kraft fat-free mayonnaise
> ½ teaspoon prepared mustard
> 1 teaspoon Worcestershire sauce
> 1 teaspoon celery seed
> ½ teaspoon paprika
> 1 tablespoon pourable Sugar Twin
> 4½ cups finely shredded cabbage

In a large bowl, combine dry milk powder, water, and 1 teaspoon vinegar. Let set for 5 minutes. Stir in mayonnaise, remaining 1 tablespoon vinegar, mustard, Worcestershire sauce, celery seed, paprika, and Sugar Twin. Add cabbage. Mix well to combine. Cover and refrigerate for at least 15 minutes. Gently stir again just before serving.

Each serving equals:

HE: 1½ Vegetable • ⅓ Skim Milk •
14 Optional Calories

56 Calories • 0 gm Fat • 3 gm Protein •
11 gm Carbohydrate • 238 mg Sodium •
122 mg Calcium • 1 gm Fiber

DIABETIC: 1 Vegetable •
½ Starch/Carbohydrate or 2 Vegetable

Oktoberfest Red Cabbage Salad

What a colorful savory salad I was able to create with these few ingredients! I give all the credit to God's own creation, red cabbage. The textures of this dish go well with hearty German dishes served at this beloved fall festival. ☻ Serves 6 (1 full cup)

> 5 cups shredded red cabbage
> 1 cup sliced fresh mushrooms
> 1½ cups frozen peas, thawed
> 6 tablespoons Dannon plain fat-free yogurt
> ⅓ cup Carnation Nonfat Dry Milk Powder
> ½ cup Kraft fat-free mayonnaise
> 2 teaspoons lemon juice
> 2 teaspoons prepared mustard
> Sugar substitute to equal ¼ cup sugar
> ⅛ teaspoon black pepper

In a large bowl, combine cabbage, mushrooms, and peas. In a medium bowl, combine yogurt and dry milk powder. Add mayonnaise, lemon juice, mustard, sugar substitute, and black pepper. Mix well to combine. Add dressing mixture to cabbage mixture. Mix gently to combine. Cover and refrigerate for at least 30 minutes. Gently stir again just before serving.

HINT: Thaw peas by placing in a colander and rinsing under hot water for one minute.

Each serving equals:

HE: 2 Vegetable • ½ Bread • ¼ Skim Milk • 17 Optional Calories

68 Calories • 0 gm Fat • 4 gm Protein • 13 gm Carbohydrate • 177 mg Sodium • 99 mg Calcium • 3 gm Fiber

DIABETIC: 1½ Vegetable • ½ Starch/Carbohydrate

Cabbage "Plus" Salad

Crunchy, sweet, and just a little tart—that's a recipe for culinary class you'll want to serve often! I always leave the skins on my apples for this kind of salad. The extra fiber and color is always welcome!   ☻   Serves 4 (1 cup)

> *2 cups shredded cabbage*
> *1 cup chopped celery*
> *1 cup (2 small) cored, unpeeled, and diced Red Delicious apples*
> *1 cup (6 ounces) seedless green grapes*
> *½ cup Kraft fat-free mayonnaise*
> *1 teaspoon lemon juice*
> *Sugar substitute to equal 2 teaspoons sugar*

In a medium bowl, combine cabbage, celery, apples, and grapes. In a small bowl, combine mayonnaise, lemon juice, and sugar substitute. Add dressing mixture to cabbage mixture. Mix well to combine. Cover and refrigerate for at least 30 minutes. Gently stir again just before serving.

Each serving equals:

HE: 1½ Vegetable • 1 Fruit • ¼ Slider • 1 Optional Calorie

80 Calories • 0 gm Fat • 1 gm Protein • 19 gm Carbohydrate • 244 mg Sodium • 35 mg Calcium • 2 gm Fiber

DIABETIC: 1 Vegetable • 1 Fruit

ABC Salad

I could say that I used this festive dish to help my grandsons learn their ABCs, but the truth is, they're so smart, they already knew them! But this salad will appeal to kids of all ages (except Cliff, who would trade this "B" for green "Beans"). It's tangy and sweet, with lots of color and crunch.   ☻   Serves 4 (1 cup)

> 1½ cups (3 small) cored, unpeeled, and diced
>   Red Delicious apples
> 1 cup chopped fresh broccoli
> 2 cups shredded cabbage
> ½ cup Kraft fat-free mayonnaise
> 1 teaspoon lemon juice
> Sugar substitute to equal 2 teaspoons sugar
> 1 teaspoon dried onion flakes

In a large bowl, combine apples, broccoli, and cabbage. In a small bowl, combine mayonnaise, lemon juice, sugar substitute, and onion flakes. Add dressing mixture to apple mixture. Mix well to combine. Cover and refrigerate for at least 30 minutes. Gently stir again just before serving.

Each serving equals:

HE: 1½ Vegetable • ¾ Fruit • ¼ Slider •
1 Optional Calorie

64 Calories • 0 gm Fat • 1 gm Protein •
15 gm Carbohydrate • 273 mg Sodium •
31 mg Calcium • 2 gm Fiber

DIABETIC: 1 Vegetable • 1 Fruit

Broccoli Harvest Salad

Whether you live on a farm or in a city where the only garden you grow is on your windowsill, please join me in celebrating the joyful harvest of good-for-you growing things! This recipe is so full of goodies, it makes wonderful party food. ☻ Serves 6 (⅔ cup)

2¾ cups chopped fresh broccoli
¼ cup raisins
1 cup (2 small) cored, unpeeled, and chopped
Red Delicious apples
¼ cup finely chopped red onion
¼ cup Hormel Bacon Bits
⅓ cup (1½ ounces) shredded Kraft reduced-fat Cheddar cheese
½ cup Kraft fat-free mayonnaise
1 tablespoon white vinegar
Sugar substitute to equal 2 teaspoons sugar

In a large bowl, combine broccoli, raisins, apples, and onion. Stir in bacon bits and Cheddar cheese. In a small bowl, combine mayonnaise, vinegar, and sugar substitute. Add dressing mixture to broccoli mixture. Mix well to combine. Cover and refrigerate for at least 20 minutes. Gently stir again just before serving.

HINT: To plump up raisins without "cooking," place in a glass measuring cup and microwave on HIGH for 20 seconds.

Each serving equals:

HE: 1 Vegetable • ⅔ Fruit • ⅓ Protein • ¼ Slider • 11 Optional Calories

94 Calories • 2 gm Fat • 5 gm Protein • 14 gm Carbohydrate • 409 mg Sodium • 70 mg Calcium • 2 gm Fiber

DIABETIC: 1 Vegetable • 1 Fruit

Creamy Cauliflower and Broccoli Salad

Someone asked me once if we get extra credit for calorie burning when we gobble down a dish like this that requires lots of crunching and chewing. Well, in a perfectly fair world, I suspect we would! The important thing here is that you're choosing to nourish yourself well, so don't focus on the calories, just on the taste.

☻ Serves 6 (1 cup)

⅓ cup Kraft Fat Free Ranch Dressing
⅔ cup Kraft fat-free mayonnaise
Sugar substitute to equal 1 teaspoon sugar
2 teaspoons dried onion flakes
¼ cup Hormel Bacon Bits
3 cups chopped fresh cauliflower
3 cups chopped fresh broccoli

In a large bowl, combine Ranch dressing, mayonnaise, and sugar substitute. Add onion flakes and bacon bits. Mix well to combine. Stir in cauliflower and broccoli. Cover and refrigerate for at least 30 minutes. Gently stir again just before serving.

Each serving equals:

HE: 2 Vegetable • ½ Slider • 16 Optional Calories

85 Calories • 1 gm Fat • 4 gm Protein •
15 gm Carbohydrate • 563 mg Sodium •
33 mg Calcium • 3 gm Fiber

DIABETIC: 1½ Vegetable • ½ Starch/Carbohydrate

Don's Cauliflower Salad

I call this "Don's" salad because I created it with my friend's taste-buds in mind, but feel free to rename it in your house after this recipe's biggest fan! Don loved digging out those little bits of bacon from the super-creamy dressing.　　◐　Serves 6 (¾ cup)

> 3 cups chopped fresh cauliflower
> ¼ cup diced green onion
> ½ cup chopped red bell pepper
> ¾ cup chopped celery
> ½ cup Kraft fat-free mayonnaise
> ⅓ cup Land O Lakes no-fat sour cream
> 1 teaspoon lemon juice
> Sugar substitute to equal 2 teaspoons sugar
> ¼ cup Hormel Bacon Bits

In a large bowl, combine cauliflower, onion, red pepper, and celery. In a small bowl, combine mayonnaise, sour cream, lemon juice, sugar substitute, and bacon bits. Add mayonnaise mixture to cauliflower mixture. Mix well to combine. Cover and refrigerate for at least 2 hours. Gently stir again just before serving.

Each serving equals:

HE: 1½ Vegetable • ½ Slider • 4 Optional Calories

69 Calories • 1 gm Fat • 4 gm Protein •
11 gm Carbohydrate • 395 mg Sodium •
41 mg Calcium • 1 gm Fiber

DIABETIC: 1 Vegetable • ½ Starch/Carbohydrate

Calico Carrot and Raisin Salad

When a recipe is called "calico," it's usually because it features a lively combination of colors and flavors, so this one is no exception. If carrot and raisin salad has begun to seem old-hat, here's a way to freshen up this favorite with some new zip and zing!

○ Serves 6 (⅔ cup)

> 2½ cups shredded carrots
> ½ cup finely chopped green bell pepper
> ½ cup raisins
> 1 cup (2 small) cored, unpeeled, and finely chopped
>   Red Delicious apples
> ½ cup Kraft fat-free mayonnaise
> 1 tablespoon cider vinegar
> Sugar substitute to equal 1 tablespoon sugar
> 1 teaspoon prepared mustard
> ¼ teaspoon celery seed

In a large bowl, combine carrots, green pepper, raisins, and apples. In a small bowl, combine mayonnaise, vinegar, sugar substitute, mustard, and celery seed. Add dressing mixture to carrot mixture. Mix gently to combine. Cover and refrigerate for at least 30 minutes. Gently stir again just before serving.

HINT: To plump up raisins without "cooking," place in a glass measuring cup and microwave on HIGH for 20 seconds.

Each serving equals:

HE: 1 Fruit • 1 Vegetable • 14 Optional Calories

88 Calories • 0 gm Fat • 1 gm Protein •
21 gm Carbohydrate • 202 mg Sodium •
23 mg Calcium • 2 gm Fiber

DIABETIC: 1 Fruit • 1 Vegetable

Carrot-Corn Combo Salad

Here's a happy blend of flavors that is especially appealing to young people, though I haven't yet met a man who didn't enjoy corn and carrots! If you never thought of stirring a bit of Brown Sugar Twin into a salad dressing, you'll be delighted at the tangy sparkle it provides in this one! ☻ Serves 4 (¾ cup)

½ cup Kraft Fat Free French Dressing
1 teaspoon dried parsley flakes
1 teaspoon prepared mustard
1 tablespoon Brown Sugar Twin
2 cups (one 16-ounce can) whole-kernel corn, rinsed and drained
1 cup (one 8-ounce can) sliced carrots, rinsed and drained
¼ cup finely chopped onion
¼ cup finely chopped green bell pepper

In a large bowl, combine French dressing, parsley flakes, mustard, and Brown Sugar Twin. Add corn, carrots, onion, and green pepper. Mix well to combine. Cover and refrigerate for at least 30 minutes. Gently stir again just before serving.

Each serving equals:

HE: 1 Bread • ¾ Vegetable • ¼ Slider •
5 Optional Calories

140 Calories • 0 gm Fat • 3 gm Protein •
32 gm Carbohydrate • 337 mg Sodium •
16 mg Calcium • 3 gm Fiber

DIABETIC: 1½ Starch • 1 Vegetable

Danish Smorgasbord Vegetable Salad

Don't you just love the word "smorgasbord"? (And not because it means a big Danish buffet where you can go crazy gobbling everything in sight!) The Danish are famous for their flavorful cold salads, and this would find a happy home in such a lively spread.

◐ Serves 4 (¾ cup)

> 2½ cups finely shredded lettuce
> ¼ cup (1 ounce) sliced ripe olives
> ¾ cup diced fresh tomatoes
> ¾ cup diced fresh mushrooms
> ½ cup chopped unpeeled cucumbers
> ½ cup Kraft Fat Free Ranch Dressing
> 2 tablespoons Kraft fat-free mayonnaise

In a large bowl, combine lettuce, olives, tomatoes, mushrooms, and cucumbers. Add Ranch dressing and mayonnaise. Mix gently to combine. Serve at once.

Each serving equals:

> HE: 2¼ Vegetable • ¼ Fat • ½ Slider •
> 5 Optional Calories
>
> ---
>
> 77 Calories • 1 gm Fat • 1 gm Protein •
> 16 gm Carbohydrate • 466 mg Sodium •
> 18 mg Calcium • 2 gm Fiber
>
> ---
>
> DIABETIC: 2 Vegetable • ½ Starch

Creamy Olde Sod Pea Salad

My friend Barbara once told me that her favorite veggie as a child was tiny peas, the one with such sweetness and delicate flavor they taste like a treat! This luscious salad takes those little delights and magnifies their flavor by blending them with chopped egg and cheese. Now that's a treat times three!

☻ Serves 12 (½ cup)

> 1½ cups Kraft fat-free mayonnaise
> ¼ cup pickle juice from a jar of bread & butter pickles
> 1 tablespoon dried onion flakes
> ¼ teaspoon black pepper
> 6 cups (three 16-ounce cans) small peas, rinsed and drained
> Scant 1½ cups (4½ ounces) cubed Healthy Choice or Velveeta
>   Light processed cheese
> 3 hard-boiled eggs, chopped

In a large bowl, combine mayonnaise, pickle juice, onion flakes, and black pepper. Add peas and cheese. Mix gently to combine. Fold in eggs. Cover and refrigerate for at least 30 minutes. Gently stir again just before serving.

Each serving equals:

HE: 1 Bread • ¾ Protein (¼ limited) • ¼ Slider

118 Calories • 2 gm Fat • 8 gm Protein •
17 gm Carbohydrate • 278 mg Sodium •
98 mg Calcium • 4 gm Fiber

DIABETIC: 1 Starch • 1 Meat

Orange-Spinach Salad

If salad has become a duty instead of a delight, here's something new to try tonight! (That rhymes—a little "kitchen poetry"!) This blends some intriguing flavors into a dish that will awaken your appetite for those good-for-you greens!

☻ Serves 4 (1 cup)

> 4 cups torn fresh spinach, stems removed and discarded
> 1 cup (one 11-ounce can) mandarin oranges, rinsed and drained
> ½ cup chopped red onion
> 1 (8-ounce) can sliced water chestnuts, drained and chopped
> ¼ cup Kraft Fat Free Honey Dijon Dressing

In a large bowl, combine spinach, mandarin oranges, onion, and water chestnuts. Add Honey Dijon dressing. Toss well to combine. Serve at once.

Each serving equals:

HE: 2¼ Vegetable • ½ Bread • ½ Fruit • ¼ Slider • 5 Optional Calories

100 Calories • 0 gm Fat • 2 gm Protein • 23 gm Carbohydrate • 382 mg Sodium • 69 mg Calcium • 4 gm Fiber

DIABETIC: 2 Vegetable • 1 Starch/Carbohydrate

Wilted Lettuce

Now, wait, I know it *sounds* like something you'd rather leave at the store than bring home, but this is a wonderful new way to serve salad. Warmed and spiced with savory dressing, the lettuce takes on a whole new pizzazz!   ☻   Serves 6 (1 cup)

> 6 cups torn leaf lettuce
> ¾ cup chopped radishes
> ½ cup Kraft Fat Free Italian Dressing
> ¼ cup Hormel Bacon Bits
> 2 teaspoons pourable Sugar Twin

In a large bowl, combine lettuce and radishes. In a small skillet, combine Italian dressing, bacon bits, and Sugar Twin. Cook over medium heat until mixture is hot, stirring often. Pour hot mixture over lettuce mixture. Quickly toss until thoroughly combined. Serve at once.

Each serving equals:

HE: 2¼ Vegetable • ¼ Slider • 11 Optional Calories

---

41 Calories • 1 gm Fat • 2 gm Protein •
6 gm Carbohydrate • 379 mg Sodium •
7 mg Calcium • 0 gm Fiber

DIABETIC: 1½ Vegetable

Fettuccine Tomato Vegetable Salad

Here's something new in a pasta salad, which just about always features shaped pastas like rotini and shells! For those of you who love these long, flat, and delicious strands of pasta, this makes a terrific pasta course served with an Italian entrée.

◐ Serves 4 (1 cup)

⅓ cup Kraft Fat Free Ranch Dressing
⅓ cup Kraft fat-free mayonnaise
¼ cup (¾ ounce) grated Kraft fat-free Parmesan cheese
⅛ teaspoon black pepper
2 cups cold cooked fettuccine, rinsed and drained
1 cup chopped fresh tomato
¾ cup chopped unpeeled cucumber
¼ cup finely chopped onion

In a large bowl, combine Ranch dressing, mayonnaise, Parmesan cheese, and black pepper. Add fettuccine. Mix well to combine. Stir in tomato, cucumber, and onion. Cover and refrigerate for at least 30 minutes. Gently stir again just before serving.

HINT: 1½ cups broken uncooked fettuccine usually cooks to about 2 cups.

Each serving equals:

HE: 1 Bread • 1 Vegetable • ¼ Protein • ½ Slider •
7 Optional Calories

173 Calories • 1 gm Fat • 5 gm Protein •
36 gm Carbohydrate • 394 mg Sodium •
12 mg Calcium • 3 gm Fiber

DIABETIC: 2 Starch/Carbohydrate • 1 Vegetable

Marinated Carrot and Rotini Salad

The magic of marinating is that letting your ingredients "hang out" together for a few hours—or even overnight—gives them the chance to mingle magnificently! It's astonishing how much difference a little extra waiting time can make, so plan ahead some evening and get this dish started in advance!

☺ Serves 8 (½ cup)

1 (10¾-ounce) can Healthy
   Request Tomato Soup
¼ cup Kraft Fat Free Italian
   Dressing
¼ cup pourable Sugar Twin
2 tablespoons white vinegar
½ teaspoon prepared mustard
1 teaspoon dried parsley flakes

2 cups (one 16-ounce can)
   sliced carrots, rinsed and
   drained
¾ cup chopped green bell
   pepper
¼ cup chopped onion
2 cups cold cooked rotini pasta,
   rinsed and drained

In a medium saucepan, combine tomato soup, Italian dressing, Sugar Twin, vinegar, mustard, and parsley flakes. Cook over medium heat until mixture starts to boil, stirring often. Remove from heat. Stir in carrots, green pepper, and onion. Add rotini pasta. Mix well to combine. Pour mixture into a large bowl. Cover and refrigerate for at least 2 hours or up to overnight. Gently stir again just before serving.

HINT: 1½ cups uncooked rotini pasta usually cooks to about 2 cups.

Each serving equals:

HE: ¾ Vegetable • ½ Bread • ¼ Slider •
11 Optional Calories

89 Calories • 1 gm Fat • 2 gm Protein •
18 gm Carbohydrate • 213 mg Sodium •
19 mg Calcium • 1 gm Fiber

DIABETIC: 1 Vegetable • 1 Starch

Family Reunion Macaroni Salad

There's just about nothing I like better than having my family gathered around me, and what better time to serve those dishes beloved by all? Macaroni salad is a great Midwestern classic, and this version is much healthier than most. Still, it delivers terrific flavor in every single bite.   ☻   Serves 8 (¾ cup)

> *4 cups cold cooked elbow macaroni, rinsed and drained*
> *1¼ cups shredded carrots*
> *¼ cup finely chopped onion*
> *½ cup finely chopped green bell pepper*
> *⅔ cup Carnation Nonfat Dry Milk Powder*
> *½ cup water*
> *½ cup Kraft fat-free mayonnaise*
> *¼ cup white vinegar*
> *⅓ cup pourable Sugar Twin*

In a large bowl, combine macaroni, carrots, onion, and green pepper. In a medium bowl, combine dry milk powder and water. Stir in mayonnaise, vinegar, and Sugar Twin. Add dressing mixture to macaroni mixture. Mix well to combine. Cover and refrigerate for at least 1 hour. Gently stir again just before serving.

HINT: 2⅔ cups uncooked elbow macaroni usually cooks to about 4 cups.

Each serving equals:

HE: 1 Bread • ½ Vegetable • ¼ Skim Milk • 14 Optional Calories

136 Calories • 0 gm Fat • 6 gm Protein • 28 gm Carbohydrate • 168 mg Sodium • 81 mg Calcium • 1 gm Fiber

DIABETIC: 1½ Starch • ½ Vegetable

Garden Glory Salad

In the 1950s, molded salads were all the rage. If I can be instrumental in bringing back tasty, pretty dishes like this one, that'd be great! It's perfect for a summer card party or festive bridal shower.

❤ Serves 6

> 1 (4-serving) package JELL-O sugar-free lemon gelatin
> ¾ cup boiling water
> ½ cup Kraft fat-free mayonnaise
> 2 cups fat-free cottage cheese
> ¾ cup shredded carrots
> ¼ cup finely chopped green bell pepper
> ½ cup finely chopped celery
> ½ cup finely chopped cucumber

In a large bowl, combine dry gelatin and boiling water. Mix well to dissolve gelatin. Place bowl on a wire rack and let set for 5 minutes, stirring occasionally. Fold in mayonnaise and cottage cheese. Add carrots, green pepper, celery, and cucumber. Mix well to combine. Pour mixture into an 8-by-8-inch dish. Refrigerate until firm, about 2 hours. Cut into 6 servings.

Each serving equals:

HE: ⅔ Protein • ⅔ Vegetable • ¼ Slider

76 Calories • 0 gm Fat • 11 gm Protein •
8 gm Carbohydrate • 505 mg Sodium •
42 mg Calcium • 0 gm Fiber

DIABETIC: 1 Meat • 1 Vegetable

Sweet Salads

All-American Apple Salad

Whether you're feeling patriotic—or you just adore apples—this is a wonderful and satisfying salad to feature on your menu! I think cheese and apples always go great together . . . just as red, white, and blue do! ☻ Serves 6 (½ cup)

⅓ cup Kraft fat-free mayonnaise
⅓ cup Land O Lakes no-fat sour cream
Sugar substitute to equal 2 teaspoons sugar
1 cup (one 8-ounce can) pineapple chunks, packed in fruit juice,
        drained, and 1 tablespoon liquid reserved ☆
2 cups (4 small) cored, unpeeled, and diced Red Delicious apples
¾ cup (3 ounces) shredded Kraft reduced-fat Cheddar cheese
¼ cup (1 ounce) chopped walnuts

In a large bowl, combine mayonnaise, sour cream, sugar substitute, and reserved pineapple juice. Add pineapple, apples, Cheddar cheese, and walnuts. Mix well to combine. Cover and refrigerate for at least 30 minutes. Gently stir again just before serving.

Each serving equals:

HE: 1 Fruit • ¾ Protein • ⅓ Fat • ¼ Slider •
8 Optional Calories

137 Calories • 5 gm Fat • 5 gm Protein •
18 gm Carbohydrate • 252 mg Sodium •
120 mg Calcium • 1 gm Fiber

DIABETIC: 1 Fruit • ½ Meat • ½ Fat

White Fruit Salad

What could be more fresh and summery than a melange of sweet fruits in the palest shades of the season? This combo looks lovely on the plate, but it's the taste that will win your family's hearts!

◑ Serves 6 (½ cup)

> 1 cup (one 8-ounce can) pineapple tidbits, packed in fruit juice, drained
> 1 cup (6 ounces) Thompson seedless grapes, halved
> 1 cup (2 small) cored and diced fresh pears
> ¼ cup (1 ounce) chopped pecans
> ½ cup (1 ounce) miniature marshmallows
> ¾ cup Cool Whip Free
> 1 teaspoon lemon juice

In a medium bowl, combine pineapple, grapes, and pears. Stir in pecans and marshmallows. Add Cool Whip Free and lemon juice. Mix gently to combine. Cover and refrigerate for at least 1 hour. Gently stir again just before serving.

HINT: If you can't find tidbits, use chunk pineapple and coarsely chop.

Each serving equals:

HE: 1 Fruit • ⅔ Fat • ¼ Slider • 3 Optional Calories

---

131 Calories • 3 gm Fat • 1 gm Protein •
25 gm Carbohydrate • 10 mg Sodium •
13 mg Calcium • 2 gm Fiber

DIABETIC: 1 Fruit • ½ Fat • ½ Starch/Carbohydrate

Blueberry Fruit Fluff Salad

Fluff is definitely "the right stuff" when it comes to pleasing the men in my life! It leaves lots of room for a hearty main dish, and the texture is just magic in your mouth! ☻ Serves 6 (⅔ cup)

> 1 (4-serving) package JELL-O sugar-free vanilla cook-and-serve pudding mix
> 1 (4-serving) package JELL-O sugar-free strawberry gelatin
> 1¼ cups water
> 1½ cups frozen unsweetened blueberries
> ¾ cup Cool Whip Free
> 1 cup (one 11-ounce can) mandarin oranges, rinsed and drained
> 1 cup (2 small) cored, unpeeled, and chopped
>   Red Delicious apples
> ¾ cup (1½ ounces) miniature marshmallows

In a medium saucepan, combine dry pudding mix, dry gelatin, and water. Stir in blueberries. Cook over medium heat until mixture thickens and starts to boil, stirring often, and being careful not to crush blueberries. Place saucepan on a wire rack and let set for 20 minutes, stirring occasionally. Spoon blueberry mixture into a large serving bowl. Stir in Cool Whip Free. Add mandarin oranges, apples, and marshmallows. Mix gently to combine. Cover and refrigerate for at least 30 minutes. Gently stir again just before serving.

Each serving equals:

HE: 1 Fruit • ½ Slider • 8 Optional Calories

---

100 Calories • 0 gm Fat • 1 gm Protein •
24 gm Carbohydrate • 125 mg Sodium •
8 mg Calcium • 1 gm Fiber

DIABETIC: 1 Fruit • ½ Starch/Carbohydrate

Blueberries and Cream Salad

They may be called *blue*berries, but when you combine them with a creamy dressing, everything turns a luscious shade of purple! The pecans add lots of crunch for very little fat and calories, so don't leave them out. ☻ Serves 8

> 2 (4-serving) packages JELL-O sugar-free cherry gelatin
> 1⅓ cups boiling water
> 1 cup Diet Mountain Dew
> 1 cup (one 8-ounce can) crushed pineapple, packed in fruit juice, undrained
> 1½ cups fresh blueberries
> ¼ cup (1 ounce) chopped pecans ☆
> ¾ cup Dannon plain fat-free yogurt
> ⅓ cup Carnation Nonfat Dry Milk Powder
> 1 teaspoon vanilla extract
> Sugar substitute to equal 2 tablespoons sugar
> 1 cup Cool Whip Free

In a large bowl, combine dry gelatins and boiling water. Mix well to dissolve gelatin. Stir in Diet Mountain Dew and undrained pineapple. Add blueberries and 2 tablespoons pecans. Mix gently to combine. Pour mixture into an 8-by-8-inch dish. Refrigerate until firm, about 3 hours. In a medium bowl, combine yogurt and dry milk powder. Stir in vanilla extract and sugar substitute. Fold in Cool Whip Free. Spread mixture evenly over set gelatin mixture. Evenly sprinkle remaining 2 tablespoons pecans over top. Refrigerate for at least 30 minutes. Cut into 8 servings.

Each serving equals:

HE: ½ Fruit • ½ Fat • ¼ Skim Milk • ¼ Slider • 6 Optional Calories

106 Calories • 2 gm Fat • 4 gm Protein • 18 gm Carbohydrate • 93 mg Sodium • 84 mg Calcium • 1 gm Fiber

DIABETIC: ½ Fruit • ½ Fat • ½ Starch/Carbohydrate

Just Plain Good Strawberry Salad

Okay, I was being modest. Anyone who knows me already knows that I think everything with strawberries is spectacular, so "just plain good" may be underselling the deliciousness of this recipe. In Iowa, this is considered a side dish, but you can also enjoy it everywhere as a light, sweet dessert! ☻ Serves 6

> 2 (4-serving) packages JELL-O sugar-free strawberry gelatin
> 1½ cups hot water
> 2 cups Wells' Blue Bunny sugar- and fat-free vanilla ice cream
>   or any sugar- and fat-free ice cream, slightly softened
> 1 (16-ounce) package frozen unsweetened strawberries

In a large bowl, combine dry gelatin and hot water. Mix well to dissolve gelatin. Add ice cream. Mix well until smooth. Stir in frozen strawberries. Pour mixture into an 8-by-8-inch dish. Refrigerate until set. Cut into 6 servings.

Each serving equals:

HE: ½ Fruit • ½ Slider • 14 Optional Calories

100 Calories • 0 gm Fat • 5 gm Protein •
20 gm Carbohydrate • 107 mg Sodium •
92 mg Calcium • 1 gm Fiber

DIABETIC: 1 Fruit • ½ Starch/Carbohydrate

Piña Colada Salad

Somewhere there's a bartender who's already earned his place in heaven by creating the fabulous tropical drink that combines pineapple and coconut so delectably! I decided to offer you those great flavors in a salad, and added a couple of surprises for good measure! ☉ Serves 6

> ¾ cup Dannon plain fat-free yogurt
> ⅓ cup Carnation Nonfat Dry Milk Powder
> 2 teaspoons coconut extract
> Sugar substitute to equal ¼ cup sugar
> ½ cup Cool Whip Free
> 1 cup (one 8-ounce can) pineapple chunks, packed in fruit juice, drained
> 1 cup (6 ounces) seedless grapes
> 2 cups sliced fresh strawberries
> 2 tablespoons flaked coconut

In a large bowl, combine yogurt and dry milk powder. Stir in coconut extract and sugar substitute. Fold in Cool Whip Free. Add pineapple, grapes, and strawberries. Mix gently to combine. Spoon mixture into 6 serving dishes. Evenly sprinkle 1 teaspoon coconut over top of each. Refrigerate for at least 30 minutes.

Each serving equals:

HE: 1 Fruit • ⅓ Skim Milk • ¼ Slider

109 Calories • 1 gm Fat • 3 gm Protein •
22 gm Carbohydrate • 51 mg Sodium •
118 mg Calcium • 1 gm Fiber

DIABETIC: 1 Fruit • ½ Starch /Carbohydrate

Heavenly Pineapple–Bing Cherry Salad

My son James is the cherry lover of the family, and he's passed that pleasure on to his sons (my grandsons!), who also adore pineapple. Boys, this was created with you in mind, because no mom or grandmom could be prouder than I am of you!

☻ Serves 8 (½ cup)

> 1 (4-serving) package JELL-O sugar-free vanilla cook-and-serve
>   pudding mix
> 1 (4-serving) package JELL-O sugar-free lemon gelatin
> 1 cup (one 8-ounce can) crushed pineapple, packed in fruit juice,
>   drained, and ⅓ cup liquid reserved ☆
> 1 cup water
> 1 cup Cool Whip Free
> 2 cups (12 ounces) bing or sweet cherries, pitted and halved
> ½ cup (1 ounce) miniature marshmallows

In a medium saucepan, combine dry pudding mix, dry gelatin, reserved pineapple liquid, and water. Cook over medium heat until mixture thickens and starts to boil, stirring often. Remove from heat. Stir in pineapple. Pour mixture into a medium bowl. Place bowl on a wire rack and let set for 20 minutes, stirring occasionally. Fold in Cool Whip Free. Add bing cherries and marshmallows. Mix gently to combine. Refrigerate for at least 30 minutes. Gently stir again just before serving.

Each serving equals:

HE: ¾ Fruit • ¼ Slider • 10 Optional Calories

84 Calories • 0 gm Fat • 1 gm Protein •
20 gm Carbohydrate • 91 mg Sodium •
10 mg Calcium • 1 gm Fiber

DIABETIC: 1 Fruit • ½ Starch/Carbohydrate

Strawberry-Lemon Gelatin Salad

How does that old song go, that sweet dreams are made of this? Well, here's a delight worthy of enjoyment day or night!

☯ Serves 8

> 1 (4-serving) package JELL-O sugar-free strawberry gelatin
>
> 1 (4-serving) package JELL-O sugar-free lemon gelatin
>
> 1 cup boiling water
>
> 1 cup Diet Mountain Dew
>
> 2 cups chopped fresh strawberries
>
> 1½ cups Dannon plain fat-free yogurt
>
> ¼ cup pourable Sugar Twin
>
> 1 teaspoon vanilla extract

In a large bowl, combine dry strawberry and lemon gelatins. Add boiling water. Mix well to dissolve gelatins. Stir in Diet Mountain Dew. Add strawberries. Mix gently to combine. Refrigerate for 45 minutes or until mixture starts to set. In a medium bowl, combine yogurt, Sugar Twin, and vanilla extract. Stir yogurt mixture into gelatin mixture. Spread mixture into an 8-by-8-inch dish. Refrigerate until firm, about 3 hours. Cut into 8 servings.

Each serving equals:

HE: ¼ Skim Milk • ¼ Fruit • 13 Optional Calories

40 Calories • 0 gm Fat • 4 gm Protein •
6 gm Carbohydrate • 91 mg Sodium •
90 mg Calcium • 0 gm Fiber

DIABETIC: ½ Starch/Carbohydrate

Lemon Delight Salad

This is one of the prettiest layered salads I've ever created, and it's definitely worth making a bit of extra time to prepare it. The actual prep time is brief (it's a Healthy Exchanges recipe, after all) but there is some waiting time between layers. I suggest an energetic walk around the neighborhood while this delicious concoction gels!   ☻   Serves 6

> 1 (4-serving) package JELL-O sugar-free
>   lemon gelatin
> 1 cup boiling water
> 1⅔ cups cold water ☆
> ½ cup (1 ounce) miniature marshmallows
> 1 cup (one 8-ounce can) crushed pineapple, packed in
>   fruit juice, drained, and ⅓ cup liquid reserved ☆
> 2 cups (2 medium) diced bananas
> 1 (4-serving) package JELL-O sugar-free vanilla
>   cook-and-serve pudding mix
> 2 teaspoons lemon juice
> 1 cup Cool Whip Free
> 2 tablespoons (½ ounce) chopped pecans

In a large bowl, combine dry gelatin and boiling water. Mix well to dissolve gelatin. Stir in 1 cup cold water. Add marshmallows, drained pineapple, and bananas. Mix well to combine. Pour mixture into an 8-by-8-inch dish. Refrigerate until firm, about 2 hours. In a medium saucepan, combine reserved pineapple liquid, remaining ⅔ cup cold water, dry pudding mix, and lemon juice. Cook over medium heat until mixture thickens and starts to boil, stirring often. Remove from heat. Place saucepan on a wire rack and allow to cool for 20 minutes, stirring occasionally. Fold in Cool Whip Free. Evenly spread mixture over gelatin mixture. Evenly sprinkle pecans over top. Refrigerate for at least 30 minutes. Cut into 6 servings.

Each serving equals:

HE: 1 Fruit • ⅓ Fat • ½ Slider • 8 Optional Calories

133 Calories • 1 gm Fat • 1 gm Protein •
30 gm Carbohydrate • 123 mg Sodium •
11 mg Calcium • 1 gm Fiber

DIABETIC: 1 Fruit • ½ Fat • ½ Starch/Carbohydrate

Pineapple Salad

It's simple, it's elegant, and its citrusy sweetness makes it a perfect accompaniment to almost any chicken or fish entrée in this book. Just make sure you keep some extra Diet Dew on hand for recipes!

☻ Serves 6

> 1 (4-serving) package JELL-O sugar-free lemon gelatin
> 1 cup boiling water
> ¾ cup Diet Mountain Dew
> ¾ cup Cool Whip Free
> 1 cup (one 8-ounce can) crushed pineapple, packed in fruit juice, drained

In a large bowl, combine dry gelatin and boiling water. Mix well to dissolve gelatin. Stir in Diet Mountain Dew. Refrigerate for 30 minutes or until mixture just starts to gel. Whip with a wire whisk until fluffy. Blend in Cool Whip Free and pineapple. Spread mixture into an 8-by-8-inch dish and refrigerate until firm, about 2 hours. Cut into 6 servings.

Each serving equals:

HE: ⅓ Fruit • ¼ Slider • 2 Optional Calories

48 Calories • 0 gm Fat • 1 gm Protein • 11 gm Carbohydrate • 45 mg Sodium • 6 mg Calcium • 0 gm Fiber

DIABETIC: ½ Fruit

Ruby Raspberry Salad

When raspberries first appear in the market or at the farm stand, it looks as if baskets of rubies are glittering in the sun! Their season isn't long, but you can make every minute of it count with this tasty, creamy salad. Get the freshest, firmest berries you can find—or grow your own! ◐ Serves 8

2 (4-serving) packages JELL-O
sugar-free raspberry gelatin
1 cup boiling water
1 cup (one 8-ounce can)
crushed pineapple, packed
in fruit juice, drained, and
¼ cup liquid reserved ☆
¾ cup cold water
1 (8-ounce) package
Philadelphia fat-free
cream cheese

¾ cup Dannon plain fat-free
yogurt
⅓ cup Carnation Nonfat Dry
Milk Powder
Sugar substitute to equal 2
tablespoons sugar
1 cup Cool Whip Free
1 teaspoon vanilla extract
1½ cups fresh red raspberries
2 tablespoons (½ ounce)
chopped pecans

In a large bowl, combine dry gelatins and boiling water. Mix well to dissolve gelatin. Stir in reserved pineapple liquid and cold water. Add cream cheese. Mix well with a wire whisk until blended. Refrigerate for 10 minutes. Meanwhile, in a small bowl, combine yogurt and dry milk powder. Add sugar substitute, Cool Whip Free, and vanilla extract. Mix gently to combine. Fold yogurt mixture into cooled gelatin mixture. Add pineapple, raspberries, and pecans. Mix gently to combine. Pour mixture into an 8-by-8-inch dish. Refrigerate for at least 2 hours. Cut into 8 servings.

Each serving equals:

HE: ½ Protein • ½ Fruit • ¼ Skim Milk • ¼ Fat •
¼ Slider • 7 Optional Calories

109 Calories • 1 gm Fat • 8 gm Protein •
17 gm Carbohydrate • 261 mg Sodium •
87 mg Calcium • 1 gm Fiber

DIABETIC: 1 Starch/Carbohydrate • ½ Meat • ½ Fruit

Tulip Time Rhubarb Salad

Some people watch for the first crocus of spring; for me, it's always the first appearance of rhubarb that tells me winter is finally over! (Of course, through the magic of flash freezing, we can enjoy rhubarb all year long. But here in Iowa, we love it best when it's fresh!) Pick a bunch of colorful tulips, then decorate your table with this! ☻ Serves 6

> *3 cups finely chopped fresh or frozen rhubarb*
> *¼ cup water*
> *⅓ cup pourable Sugar Twin*
> *1 (4-serving) package JELL-O sugar-free strawberry gelatin*
> *1 cup unsweetened orange juice*
> *1 cup sliced fresh strawberries*

In a medium saucepan, combine rhubarb, water, and Sugar Twin. Cover and cook over medium heat for 10 minutes or until rhubarb becomes soft, stirring occasionally. Remove from heat. Add dry gelatin and orange juice. Mix well to dissolve gelatin. Stir in strawberries. Pour mixture into an 8-by-8-inch dish. Refrigerate until firm, about 3 hours. Cut into 6 servings.

Each serving equals:

HE: 1 Vegetable • ½ Fruit • 12 Optional Calories

---

44 Calories • 0 gm Fat • 2 gm Protein •
9 gm Carbohydrate • 40 mg Sodium •
59 mg Calcium • 1 gm Fiber

DIABETIC: 1 Vegetable • ½ Fruit

Vegetables

Baked Asparagus in Egg Sauce

When I was growing up, we used to think of asparagus as kind of a luxury food—something to enjoy only on special occasions. Now, it's just one of the many vegetables we can relish anytime at all—and this recipe turns it into a star!   ☺   Serves 4

> ¼ cup chopped onion
> 1 (10¾-ounce) can Healthy Request Cream of Celery Soup
> ⅓ cup Carnation Nonfat Dry Milk Powder
> ¼ cup water
> 2 teaspoons lemon juice
> 2 hard-boiled eggs, chopped
> 1¾ cups (one 14.5-ounce can) cut asparagus, rinsed and drained
> 9 tablespoons (2¼ ounces) dried fine bread crumbs

Preheat oven to 350 degrees. Spray an 8-by-8-inch baking dish with butter-flavored cooking spray. In a large skillet sprayed with butter-flavored cooking spray, sauté onion for 5 minutes. Stir in celery soup, dry milk powder, water, and lemon juice. Continue cooking for 5 minutes, stirring occasionally. Add eggs. Mix gently to combine. Remove from heat. Evenly arrange asparagus in prepared baking dish. Spoon soup mixture evenly over asparagus. Evenly sprinkle bread crumbs over top. Lightly spray crumbs with butter-flavored cooking spray. Bake for 25 to 30 minutes or until casserole is bubbly and crumbs are browned. Place baking dish on a wire rack and let set for 5 minutes. Divide into 4 servings.

Each serving equals:

HE: 1 Vegetable • ¾ Bread • ½ Protein (limited) • ¼ Skim Milk • ½ Slider • 1 Optional Calorie

187 Calories • 7 gm Fat • 9 gm Protein • 22 gm Carbohydrate • 762 mg Sodium • 152 mg Calcium • 2 gm Fiber

DIABETIC: 1 Vegetable • 1 Starch • ½ Meat • ½ Fat

Celery au Gratin

When a classic veggie like celery takes center stage, as it does here, you may be surprised to discover just how delicious it can be! This side dish is so spectacular, it's delightful served at a festive dinner party for good friends.   ☻   Serves 6

4½ cups chopped celery

1½ cups water

1½ cups (one 12-fluid-ounce can) Carnation Evaporated Skim Milk

¼ cup all-purpose flour

¼ cup (one 2-ounce jar) chopped pimiento, drained

1 teaspoon lemon pepper

1 (7.5-ounce) can Pillsbury refrigerated buttermilk biscuits

⅓ cup (1½ ounces) shredded Kraft reduced-fat Cheddar cheese

Preheat oven to 375 degrees. Spray an 8-by-8-inch baking dish with butter-flavored cooking spray. In a medium saucepan, cook celery in water for 8 to 10 minutes or just until tender. Drain well. In a covered jar, combine evaporated skim milk and flour. Shake well to blend. Pour milk mixture into same saucepan, now sprayed with butter-flavored cooking spray. Cook over medium heat until mixture thickens and starts to boil, stirring constantly. Stir in drained celery, pimiento, and lemon pepper. Pour celery mixture into prepared baking dish. Cut each biscuit into 4 pieces. Evenly arrange biscuit pieces over celery mixture. Sprinkle Cheddar cheese evenly over top. Bake for 20 to 25 minutes. Place baking dish on a wire rack and let set for 5 minutes. Divide into 6 servings.

Each serving equals:

HE: 1½ Bread • 1½ Vegetable • ½ Skim Milk • ⅓ Protein

203 Calories • 3 gm Fat • 10 gm Protein • 34 gm Carbohydrate • 486 mg Sodium • 264 mg Calcium • 3 gm Fiber

DIABETIC: 1½ Starch • 1 Vegetable • ½ Skim Milk • ½ Fat

Skillet Cabbage

This is a true example of easy culinary magic—just a few common ingredients and only minutes in the kitchen produces a flavorful, high-fiber accompaniment that will perk up everyone's tastebuds!

○ Serves 4 (¾ cup)

> 2 tablespoons Kraft Fat Free Italian Dressing
> 3 cups shredded cabbage
> 1 cup chopped celery
> ½ cup chopped green bell pepper
> ½ cup chopped onion
> ⅛ teaspoon black pepper

Pour Italian dressing into a large skillet. Cook over medium heat for 3 to 5 minutes or until dressing is hot. Stir in cabbage, celery, green pepper, onion, and black pepper. Cover and continue cooking for 6 to 8 minutes, or until vegetables are tender, stirring occasionally.

Each serving equals:

HE: 2½ Vegetable • 4 Optional Calories

32 Calories • 0 gm Fat • 1 gm Protein • 7 gm Carbohydrate • 114 mg Sodium • 42 mg Calcium • 2 gm Fiber

DIABETIC: 1½ Vegetable

Grecian Green Beans

Whenever I do a cooking demonstration, I bring along my favorite preparation bowl—an 8-cup glass measuring cup! Besides being perfect for stirring up pies and other goodies, it's also just right for cooking up a simply delectable veggie dish in your microwave!

☻ Serves 4 (½ cup)

3 cups fresh or frozen cut green beans
2 tablespoons water
¼ cup (1 ounce) chopped walnuts
⅓ cup (1½ ounces) crumbled feta cheese

In an 8-cup glass measuring bowl, combine green beans and water. Cover and microwave on HIGH (100% power) for 10 to 12 minutes or just until green beans are tender, stirring after 5 minutes. Drain well and return to bowl. Stir in walnuts and feta cheese. Continue to microwave on HIGH for 1 to 2 minutes. Stir well before serving.

Each serving equals:

HE: 1½ Vegetable • ¾ Protein • ½ Fat

129 Calories • 9 gm Fat • 4 gm Protein • 8 gm Carbohydrate • 229 mg Sodium • 125 mg Calcium • 1 gm Fiber

DIABETIC: 1½ Vegetable • ½ Meat • ½ Fat

Green Bean Bake

I probably have more recipes featuring green beans than any other vegetable. The reason? My husband, Cliff, the truck drivin' man, gives them the number one spot on his list of favorites. Creating tasty, healthy food for the people you love is especially satisfying—you're filling their tummies *and* satisfying their souls!   ☻   Serves 6

> 1 (10¾-ounce) can Healthy Request Cream of Mushroom Soup
> ½ cup skim milk
> 1 teaspoon Worcestershire sauce
> ⅛ teaspoon black pepper
> 15 Ritz Reduced Fat Crackers ☆
> 2 tablespoons dried onion flakes ☆
> 4 cups (two 16-ounce cans) cut green beans, rinsed and drained
> ½ cup (one 2.5-ounce jar) sliced mushrooms, drained

Preheat oven to 350 degrees. Spray an 8-by-8-inch baking dish with butter-flavored cooking spray. In a large bowl, combine mushroom soup, skim milk, Worcestershire sauce, and black pepper. Crush 5 crackers. Stir crushed crackers and 1 tablespoon onion flakes into soup mixture. Add green beans and mushrooms. Mix well to combine. Spread mixture into prepared baking dish. Crush remaining 10 crackers. In a small bowl, combine cracker crumbs and remaining 1 tablespoon onion flakes. Evenly sprinkle crumb mixture over top. Bake for 25 to 30 minutes or until mixture is hot and bubbly. Place baking dish on a wire rack and let set for 5 minutes. Divide into 6 servings.

HINT: A self-seal sandwich bag works great for crushing crackers.

Each serving equals:

HE: 1½ Vegetable • ½ Bread • ¼ Slider •
18 Optional Calories

94 Calories • 2 gm Fat • 3 gm Protein •
16 gm Carbohydrate • 300 mg Sodium •
53 mg Calcium • 1 gm Fiber

DIABETIC: 1½ Vegetable • ½ Starch

Baked Eggplant

It's one of the most beautiful vegetables you'll ever see, but many people tell me they don't always know what to do with this purple-skinned creation! Here's one of my favorite, family-pleasing ways to serve it.   ☻   Serves 6

> 3 cups peeled and diced eggplant
> ¼ cup finely chopped onion
> 2 cups water
> 1¾ cups (one 14½-ounce can) stewed tomatoes, undrained
> 1 cup (28 small) crushed fat-free saltine crackers
> 2 tablespoons Hormel Bacon Bits
> 1 tablespoon pourable Sugar Twin
> ⅛ teaspoon black pepper

Preheat oven to 350 degrees. Spray an 8-by-8-inch baking dish with butter-flavored cooking spray. In a large saucepan, combine eggplant and onion. Cover with water. Cook over medium heat for 8 to 10 minutes or until eggplant is tender. Drain thoroughly. Return vegetables to saucepan and mash well with a potato masher or fork. Add undrained stewed tomatoes, cracker crumbs, bacon bits, Sugar Twin, and black pepper. Mix well to combine. Spread mixture evenly into prepared baking dish. Bake for 45 minutes. Place baking dish on a wire rack and let set for 5 minutes. Divide into 6 servings.

HINT: A self-seal sandwich bag works great for crushing crackers.

Each serving equals:

HE: 1⅔ Vegetable • ⅔ Bread • 10 Optional Calories

98 Calories • 2 gm Fat • 3 gm Protein •
17 gm Carbohydrate • 477 mg Sodium •
58 mg Calcium • 2 gm Fiber

DIABETIC: 2 Vegetable • ½ Starch

Eggplant Parmesan

This is the way most people have enjoyed eggplant in restaurants, but unfortunately, the traditional way of preparing it is loaded with oil. It took some ingenuity and investigation to make it still taste yummy without all that fat, but I think you'll agree I've done it.

○ Serves 4

> 6 tablespoons (1½ ounces) dried fine bread crumbs
> ¼ cup (¾ ounce) grated Kraft fat-free Parmesan cheese
> 2 tablespoons Kraft Fat Free Italian Dressing
> 1¾ cups (one 15-ounce can) Hunt's Tomato Sauce
> 1 teaspoon Italian Seasoning
> 2 teaspoons pourable Sugar Twin
> 3 cups peeled and diced eggplant
> 1½ cups (6 ounces) shredded Kraft reduced-fat mozzarella cheese

Preheat oven to 350 degrees. Spray an 8-by-8-inch baking dish with olive oil–flavored cooking spray. In a small bowl, combine bread crumbs, Parmesan cheese, and Italian dressing. In another small bowl, combine tomato sauce, Italian seasoning, and Sugar Twin. Spoon ¼ cup tomato sauce mixture into prepared baking dish. Layer half of eggplant over sauce. Sprinkle half of crumb mixture over eggplant. Spoon half of tomato sauce mixture over top. Repeat layers. Evenly sprinkle mozzarella cheese over top. Bake for 35 to 40 minutes, or until eggplant is tender. Place baking dish on a wire rack and let set for 5 minutes. Divide into 4 servings.

Each serving equals:

HE: 3¼ Vegetable • 2¼ Protein • ½ Bread • 6 Optional Calories

248 Calories • 8 gm Fat • 17 gm Protein • 27 gm Carbohydrate • 990 mg Sodium • 340 mg Calcium • 6 gm Fiber

DIABETIC: 3 Vegetable • 2 Meat • ½ Starch

Mozzarella Italian Stewed Tomatoes

Here's a scrumptious dish that couldn't be simpler, but that delivers so much cozy goodness, you'll serve it often! It's even good if the bread is just a little bit stale, because it'll soften up beautifully in cooking .   ❂   Serves 4 (½ cup)

1¾ cups (one 14½-ounce can) stewed tomatoes, undrained
¼ cup chopped onion
1 teaspoon Italian seasoning
2 slices reduced-calorie Italian bread, torn into pieces
¾ cup (3 ounces) shredded Kraft reduced-fat mozzarella cheese

In an 8-cup glass measuring bowl, combine undrained stewed tomatoes, onion, and Italian seasoning. Add bread and mozzarella cheese. Mix well to combine. Microwave on HIGH (100% power) for 5 to 6 minutes or until cheese melts, stirring after 3 minutes. Let set 1 to 2 minutes before serving.

Each serving equals:

HE: 1 Protein • 1 Vegetable • ¼ Bread

120 Calories • 4 gm Fat • 9 gm Protein •
12 gm Carbohydrate • 530 mg Sodium •
221 mg Calcium • 2 gm Fiber

DIABETIC: 1 Meat • 1 Vegetable • ½ Starch

Dill Dumplings in Stewed Tomatoes

I've become such a fan of dill now that my garden produces more than any three cooks could ever use! In this recipe, I recommend the dried dill weed, since not every cook grows her own at home. These look just lovely and take very little work to make!

☯ Serves 4 (1 dumpling and ¾ cup tomato mixture)

> 3½ cups (two 14½-ounce cans) stewed tomatoes, undrained
> ¾ cup Bisquick Reduced Fat Baking Mix
> ½ teaspoon dried dill weed
> 1 tablespoon pourable Sugar Twin
> ½ cup skim milk
> ¼ cup Land O Lakes no-fat sour cream

In a large skillet sprayed with butter-flavored cooking spray, heat undrained stewed tomatoes to boiling, stirring occasionally. Meanwhile, in a medium bowl, combine baking mix, dill weed, and Sugar Twin. Add skim milk and sour cream. Mix well to combine. Drop by tablespoon into boiling stewed tomatoes to form 4 dumplings. Lower heat, cover, and simmer for 10 minutes, or until dumplings are tender.

Each serving equals:

> HE: 1¾ Vegetable • 1 Bread • ¼ Slider •
> 8 Optional Calories

> 157 Calories • 1 gm Fat • 5 gm Protein •
> 32 gm Carbohydrate • 927 mg Sodium •
> 182 mg Calcium • 2 gm Fiber

> DIABETIC: 2 Vegetable • 1½ Starch/Carbohydrate

Kitchen Vegetable Medley

Oh, dear, you've having guests for dinner and your main dish is just about ready, but you forgot to make a side dish—what can you do? Here's my trusty, last-minute solution that will save the day again and again. I bet you've got the ingredients in the pantry, and as long as you never run out of lemon pepper, you're all set!

○ Serves 4 (¾ cup)

> 2 cups (one 16-ounce can) sliced carrots, rinsed and drained
> 2 cups (one 16-ounce can) cut green beans, rinsed and drained
> ½ cup (one 2.5-ounce jar) sliced mushrooms, undrained
> 2 teaspoons lemon pepper

In a medium saucepan, combine carrots, green beans, undrained mushrooms, and lemon pepper. Cover and simmer for 10 minutes, or until mixture is heated through, stirring occasionally.

Each serving equals:

HE: 2¼ Vegetable

36 Calories • 0 gm Fat • 1 gm Protein •
8 gm Carbohydrate • 82 mg Sodium •
36 mg Calcium • 2 gm Fiber

DIABETIC: 2 Vegetable

Easy Vegetables Alfredo

Just about everyone trying to eat healthy has eliminated the word "Alfredo" from the menu, since that creamy, cheesy preparation has earned a terrible reputation for its high fat and loads of calories. Well, cheer up—Alfredo's back, and you've got him! This version is utterly convincing—and impossible to resist!

◐ Serves 4 (1 scant cup)

> 4 cups frozen carrot, broccoli, and cauliflower blend,
>   partially thawed
> 2 tablespoons water
> 1 (10¾-ounce) can Healthy Request Cream of Mushroom Soup
> ¼ cup (¾ ounce) grated Kraft fat-free Parmesan cheese
> 1 teaspoon dried parsley flakes

In an 8-cup glass measuring bowl, combine vegetable blend and water. Cover and microwave on HIGH (100% power) for 10 minutes or until vegetables are tender. Add mushroom soup, Parmesan cheese, and parsley flakes. Mix well to combine. Re-cover and continue to microwave on HIGH for 2 minutes or until mixture is hot and bubbly.

HINT: Good served over hot noodles or spaghetti.

Each serving equals:

HE: 2 Vegetable • ¼ Protein • ½ Slider •
1 Optional Calorie

110 Calories • 2 gm Fat • 5 gm Protein •
18 gm Carbohydrate • 484 mg Sodium •
99 mg Calcium • 4 gm Fiber

DIABETIC: 2 Vegetable • ½ Starch

Zucchini with Corn

I'm a big fan of "cooking" with ready-made dressing. It's one of the tricks no busy cook can afford to ignore. This recipe is a perfect example of how a few handy ingredients blended together in a skillet make an everyday dinner feel like a special treat!

◐ Serves 2 (1 cup)

2 tablespoons Kraft Fat Free Italian Dressing
1½ cups chopped zucchini
½ cup chopped onion
1 cup (one 8-ounce can) whole-kernel corn, rinsed and drained
¼ cup (one 2-ounce jar) chopped pimiento, drained

In a large skillet, combine Italian dressing, zucchini, and onion. Cook over medium heat for 5 minutes or until vegetables are tender, stirring often. Stir in corn and pimiento. Continue cooking for 2 to 3 minutes or until mixture is heated through, stirring occasionally.

Each serving equals:

HE: 2 Vegetable • 1 Bread • 8 Optional Calories

112 Calories • 0 gm Fat • 4 gm Protein •
24 gm Carbohydrate • 165 mg Sodium •
25 mg Calcium • 4 gm Fiber

DIABETIC: 2 Vegetable • 1 Starch

Creamy Succotash

This unusual-sounding name comes from Native American tradition, and in its most basic recipe usually combines lima beans and corn. I thought it would be fun to go a step or two further, and stir up a dish that just shimmers with heartwarming flavors. This luscious, cheesy blend is the result! ☻ Serves 6 (1 cup)

3 cups frozen whole-kernel corn, thawed
3 cups frozen cut green beans, thawed
3 cups frozen green lima beans, thawed
1 cup chopped onion
1½ cups chopped celery
1 (10¾-ounce) can Healthy Request Cream of Celery soup
¾ cup (3 ounces) shredded Kraft reduced-fat Cheddar cheese
½ teaspoon dried basil
⅛ teaspoon black pepper

In a slow cooker container, combine corn, green beans, lima beans, onion, and celery. Stir in celery soup. Add Cheddar cheese, basil, and black pepper. Mix well to combine. Cover and cook on LOW for 6 to 8 hours. Stir well before serving.

Each serving equals:

HE: 2½ Vegetable • 1 Bread • ⅔ Protein • ¼ Slider •
8 Optional Calories

155 Calories • 3 gm Fat • 8 gm Protein •
24 gm Carbohydrate • 273 mg Sodium •
140 mg Calcium • 5 gm Fiber

DIABETIC: 1½ Vegetable • 1 Starch • ½ Meat

Baked Corn with Mushrooms

Men just love creamed corn, I've discovered, and this recipe will easily win their hearts with just a mouthful! I've created lots of corn casseroles, but the crunchy topping and mushroom slices really make this one special. ☻ Serves 6

> 2 cups (one 16-ounce can) cream-style corn
> ¼ cup finely diced onion
> 1 (10¾-ounce) can Healthy Request Cream of Mushroom Soup
> ½ cup (one 2.5-ounce jar) sliced mushrooms
> 1 cup (1½ ounces) crushed cornflakes
> ⅛ teaspoon black pepper

Preheat oven to 350 degrees. Spray an 8-by-8-inch baking dish with butter-flavored cooking spray. In a medium bowl, combine corn, onion, mushroom soup, and mushrooms. Add cornflakes and black pepper. Mix gently to combine. Pour mixture into prepared baking dish. Bake for 45 minutes. Place baking dish on a wire rack and let set for 5 minutes. Divide into 6 servings.

Each serving equals:

HE: 1 Bread • ¼ Vegetable • ¼ Slider •
8 Optional Calories

113 Calories • 1 gm Fat • 2 gm Protein •
24 gm Carbohydrate • 541 mg Sodium •
39 mg Calcium • 2 gm Fiber

DIABETIC: 1½ Starch

Heartland Corn and Beans

Cliff and I spend a lot of each year on the road promoting Healthy Exchanges and my cookbooks, so it's a comfort to return home to Iowa each time and enjoy a dinner that reminds us how good it feels to be back. This dish celebrates the state we love and flavors that just say welcome! ☯ Serves 4 (1 cup)

> 3 cups frozen cut green beans
> ½ cup finely chopped onion
> 1 full cup (6 ounces) diced Dubuque 97% fat-free ham or any
>   extra-lean ham
> 1 cup (5 ounces) diced raw potatoes
> 2 cups water
> 1½ cups frozen whole-kernel corn
> ⅛ teaspoon black pepper

In a large skillet, combine green beans, onion, ham, potatoes, and water. Cover and cook over medium-low heat for 30 minutes or just until vegetables are tender. Stir in corn and black pepper. Lower heat and simmer for 10 minutes, or until corn is tender and most of water is evaporated, stirring occasionally.

HINT: When in season, try substituting fresh vegetables for frozen.

Each serving equals:

HE: 1¾ Vegetable • 1 Bread • 1 Protein •

145 Calories • 1 gm Fat • 10 gm Protein •
24 gm Carbohydrate • 367 mg Sodium •
34 mg Calcium • 3 gm Fiber

DIABETIC: 1½ Vegetable • 1 Starch • 1 Meat

Orange-Glazed Peas and Mushrooms

I got a few surprised looks when we were testing this recipe, but the smiles that followed every spoonful proved to me I'd hit on a winner! I think it works because the orange flavor is both tart and sweet all at once. Enjoy! ☻ Serves 4 (½ cup)

3 tablespoons orange marmalade spreadable fruit
1 tablespoon + 1 teaspoon reduced-calorie margarine
½ cup sliced fresh mushrooms
2 cups frozen peas, thawed

In a large skillet sprayed with butter-flavored cooking spray, combine spreadable fruit and margarine. Stir in mushrooms. Cook over medium heat just until mushrooms are tender, stirring often. Add peas. Mix well to combine. Lower heat and simmer for 5 minutes, or until mixture is heated through, stirring occasionally.

HINT: Thaw peas by placing in a colander and rinsing under hot water for one minute.

Each serving equals:

HE: 1 Bread • ¾ Fruit • ½ Fat • ¼ Vegetable

97 Calories • 1 gm Fat • 4 gm Protein •
18 gm Carbohydrate • 22 mg Sodium •
18 mg Calcium • 4 gm Fiber

DIABETIC: 1 Starch • ½ Fruit • ½ Fat

Lima Bean Bake

If you weren't a big fan of lima beans as a kid, it's definitely time to give them a second chance! The smoky-rich taste of this dish makes it a great accompaniment to your favorite meaty supper, especially pork. Cliff gobbled his down with a satisfied grin, so I knew I'd "done good!"   ☻   Serves 6

> ½ cup chopped onion
> ½ cup chopped green bell pepper
> 1 cup (one 8-ounce can) Hunt's Tomato Sauce
> 2 tablespoons Brown Sugar Twin
> 2 tablespoons pourable Sugar Twin
> 1 teaspoon Worcestershire sauce
> 30 ounces (three 16-ounce cans) butter or lima beans,
>   rinsed and drained
> 2 tablespoons Hormel Bacon Bits

Preheat oven to 375 degrees. Spray an 8-by-8-inch baking dish with butter-flavored cooking spray. In a large skillet sprayed with butter-flavored cooking spray, sauté onion and green pepper just until tender. Stir in tomato sauce, Brown Sugar Twin, Sugar Twin, and Worcestershire sauce. Add lima beans and bacon bits. Mix well to combine. Pour mixture into prepared baking dish. Bake for 1 hour. Place baking dish on a wire rack and let set for 5 minutes. Divide into 6 servings.

Each serving equals:

HE: 2½ Protein • 1 Vegetable • 12 Optional Calories

193 Calories • 1 gm Fat • 12 gm Protein •
34 gm Carbohydrate • 363 mg Sodium •
29 mg Calcium • 11 gm Fiber

DIABETIC: 1½ Starch • 1 Meat • 1 Vegetable

Secret Skillet Potatoes

I could have kept this scrumptious dish all to myself, but when it comes to sharing healthy kitchen secrets, I've got "loose lips!" I especially recommend this recipe to all those "non-cook cooks" out there. You'll feel like a prize-winning chef in no time!

○   Serves 4 (¾ cup)

> ½ cup Kraft Fat Free Italian Dressing
> ½ cup chopped onion
> 4½ cups (15 ounces) frozen loose-packed hash browns
> ¾ cup (3 ounces) shredded Kraft reduced-fat Cheddar cheese

In a large skillet, combine Italian dressing and onion. Stir in hash browns. Cook over medium heat for 10 minutes, stirring often. Add Cheddar cheese. Mix well to combine. Lower heat, cover, and simmer for 5 minutes, stirring occasionally.

Each serving equals:

HE: 1 Protein • ¾ Bread • ¼ Vegetable • 16 Optional Calories

156 Calories • 4 gm Fat • 7 gm Protein • 23 gm Carbohydrate • 506 mg Sodium • 157 mg Calcium • 2 gm Fiber

DIABETIC: 1 Meat • 1 Starch

Main Dishes

Tomato-Broccoli Fettuccine

You don't have to go out for a special Italian meal tonight—instead, enjoy a fresh and appealing pasta entree right at your own dinner table! This tastes luxurious and looks as if you fussed for hours, but only you know how quick and easy it really was!

○ Serves 4 (1 full cup)

1 cup chopped fresh broccoli

1 (10¾-ounce) can Healthy Request Cream of Broccoli Soup

¾ cup (3 ounces) shredded Kraft reduced-fat Cheddar cheese

¼ cup (¾ ounce) grated Kraft fat-free Parmesan cheese

½ cup skim milk

1 teaspoon dried basil

2 cups hot cooked fettuccine, rinsed and drained

1 cup peeled and chopped fresh tomato

In a large skillet sprayed with butter-flavored cooking spray, sauté broccoli for 5 minutes. Stir in broccoli soup, Cheddar cheese, Parmesan cheese, and skim milk. Cook over medium heat for 6 to 8 minutes or until cheeses melt, stirring often. Add basil, fettuccine, and tomato. Mix well to combine. Lower heat and simmer for 5 minutes, stirring occasionally.

HINT: 1½ cups broken uncooked fettuccine usually cooks to about 2 cups.

Each serving equals:

HE: 1¼ Protein • 1 Bread • 1 Vegetable • ½ Slider • 1 Optional Calorie

264 Calories • 8 gm Fat • 14 gm Protein • 34 gm Carbohydrate • 581 mg Sodium • 285 mg Calcium • 3 gm Fiber

DIABETIC: 1½ Starch • 1 Meat • ½ Vegetable

Italian Broccoli Noodle Casserole ✻

I'm a big fan of fresh broccoli, but I always keep packages of frozen broccoli on hand for recipes like this one. It's a great example of how a small amount of reduced-fat cheeses can deliver a BIG wallop of taste!   ☻   Serves 4 (1 full cup)

> 1 (10¾-ounce) can Healthy Request Cream of Mushroom Soup
> ¼ cup Kraft Fat Free Italian Dressing
> ¼ cup water
> ¾ cup (3 ounces) shredded Kraft reduced-fat mozzarella cheese
> ¼ cup (¾ ounce) grated Kraft fat-free Parmesan cheese
> 3 cups frozen cut broccoli, thawed
> 1¾ cups (3 ounces) uncooked noodles
> ½ cup finely chopped onion

In a slow cooker container, combine mushroom soup, Italian dressing, water, mozzarella cheese, and Parmesan cheese. Add broccoli, uncooked noodles, and onion. Mix well to combine. Cover and cook on LOW for 6 to 8 hours. Mix well just before serving.

Each serving equals:

HE: 1¾ Vegetable • 1¼ Protein • 1 Bread •
½ Slider • 1 Optional Calorie

250 Calories • 6 gm Fat • 13 gm Protein •
36 gm Carbohydrate • 698 mg Sodium •
233 mg Calcium • 4 gm Fiber

DIABETIC: 2 Vegetable • 1½ Starch • 1 Meat

Broccoli Alfredo

My daughter-in-law Pam, hard-working mom of three boys (!), has always loved Alfredo-type dishes, so I asked for her opinion when I was stirring this one up. Once I saw her satisfied smile, I knew this recipe would please everyone who loves such creamy-sauced pasta!

☻ Serves 4

⅓ cup Carnation Nonfat Dry Milk Powder
½ cup hot water
½ cup (1½ ounces) grated Kraft fat-free Parmesan cheese
½ cup (4 ounces) Philadelphia fat-free cream cheese
½ teaspoon dried minced garlic
2 cups frozen cut broccoli, thawed
2 cups hot cooked fettuccine, rinsed and drained

In a large skillet sprayed with butter-flavored cooking spray, combine dry milk powder, water, Parmesan cheese, cream cheese, and garlic. Cook over medium heat for 5 minutes or until mixture is smooth, stirring often. Add broccoli and fettuccine. Mix well to combine. Lower heat and simmer for 15 minutes or until mixture is heated through, stirring occasionally.

HINTS: 1. Thaw broccoli by placing in a colander and rinsing under hot water for one minute.
2. 1½ cups uncooked fettuccine usually cooks to about 2 cups.

Each serving equals:

HE: 1 Bread • 1 Protein • 1 Vegetable • ¼ Skim Milk

185 Calories • 1 gm Fat • 12 gm Protein •
32 gm Carbohydrate • 373 mg Sodium •
96 mg Calcium • 3 gm Fiber

DIABETIC: 1½ Starch • 1 Vegetable • 1 Meat

Walnut and Garlic Linguine

I get many of my best ideas while we're on the road, because Cliff and I eat dinner in so many different restaurants in so many different parts of the country. I saw this on a menu and thought, "What an interesting combination of ingredients!" The garlic isn't overwhelming, just fragrant and flavorful, and the walnuts provide a wonderful boost of texture and taste. ● Serves 4 (¾ cup)

> ⅔ cup warm water
> ⅓ cup Carnation Nonfat Dry Milk Powder
> ½ teaspoon dried minced garlic
> 1 teaspoon dried basil
> ½ teaspoon dried parsley flakes
> ¼ cup (¾ ounce) grated Kraft fat-free Parmesan cheese
> 2 cups hot cooked linguine or spaghetti, rinsed and drained
> ¼ cup (1 ounce) chopped walnuts

In a large skillet sprayed with butter-flavored cooking spray, combine water, dry milk powder, garlic, basil, and parsley flakes. Add Parmesan cheese. Mix well to combine. Stir in linguine and walnuts. Cook over medium heat for 10 minutes or until mixture is heated through, stirring often.

HINT: 1½ cups broken uncooked linguine usually cooks to about 2 cups.

Each serving equals:

HE: 1 Bread • ½ Protein • ½ Fat • ¼ Skim Milk

---

181 Calories • 5 gm Fat • 7 gm Protein • 27 gm Carbohydrate • 112 mg Sodium • 81 mg Calcium • 2 gm Fiber

---

DIABETIC: 1 Starch • 1 Fat • ½ Meat

Grande Baked Spaghetti

I think the concept of baked spaghetti may be a Midwestern tradition, but I've done my best to share this hearty pasta dish with the rest of the country through my recipes. This version is just spicy enough to tickle your tastebuds, and simple to stir up on a night when you're rushed. Olé!   ☻   Serves 6

> 1½ cups chopped unpeeled zucchini
> ½ cup chopped red bell pepper
> 1¾ cups (one 15-ounce can) Hunt's Tomato Sauce
> ½ cup chunky salsa (mild, medium, or hot)
> 1 teaspoon chili seasoning
> 3 cups hot cooked spaghetti, rinsed and drained
> 1½ cups (6 ounces) shredded Kraft reduced-fat Cheddar cheese ☆

Preheat oven to 350 degrees. Spray an 8-by-12-inch baking dish with olive oil–flavored cooking spray. In a large skillet sprayed with olive oil–flavored cooking spray, sauté zucchini and red pepper for 5 minutes or until vegetables are just tender. Add tomato sauce, salsa, and chili seasoning. Mix well to combine. Stir in spaghetti and 1 cup Cheddar cheese. Spread mixture evenly into prepared baking dish. Evenly sprinkle remaining ½ cup Cheddar cheese over top. Bake for 25 to 30 minutes. Place baking dish on a wire rack and let set for 5 minutes. Divide into 6 servings.

HINT: 2½ cups broken uncooked spaghetti usually cooks to about 3 cups.

Each serving equals:

HE: 2 Vegetable • 1⅓ Protein • 1 Bread

---

201 Calories • 5 gm Fat • 12 gm Protein • 27 gm Carbohydrate • 780 mg Sodium • 225 mg Calcium • 3 gm Fiber

---

DIABETIC: 2 Vegetable • 1 Meat • 1 Starch

Fresh Tomato Pie

If you're lucky enough to have a productive tomato patch, then this recipe just might become a weekly staple of your summer menus! I've always enjoyed tomatoes in every form, but there's something especially delectable about using the ripest, reddest, fresh-from-the-garden tomatoes.   ☻   Serves 6

1½ cups (2¼ ounces) unseasoned dry bread cubes ☆
2½ cups peeled and sliced fresh tomatoes ☆
½ cup chopped onion ☆
1 cup + 2 tablespoons (4½ ounces) shredded Kraft reduced-fat
    Cheddar cheese ☆
2 eggs, slightly beaten, or equivalent in egg substitute
1 tablespoon pourable Sugar Twin
½ teaspoon lemon pepper
2 tablespoons Hormel Bacon Bits
2 teaspoons dried parsley flakes

Preheat oven to 350 degrees. Spray a deep-dish 10-inch pie plate with butter-flavored cooking spray. Cover bottom of pie plate with 1 cup bread cubes. Layer 1½ cups tomatoes, ¼ cup onion, and ¾ cup Cheddar cheese over top. Repeat layers for tomato, onion, and cheese. In a small bowl, combine eggs, Sugar Twin, lemon pepper, bacon bits, and parsley flakes. Spoon egg mixture evenly over cheese. Evenly sprinkle remaining ½ cup bread cubes over top. Lightly spray top with butter-flavored cooking spray. Bake for 45 to 50 minutes. Place pie plate on a wire rack and let set for 5 minutes. Cut into 6 servings.

Each serving equals:

HE: 1⅓ Protein (⅓ limited) • 1 Vegetable • ½ Bread •
1 Optional Calorie

158 Calories • 6 gm Fat • 11 gm Protein •
15 gm Carbohydrate • 417 mg Sodium •
157 mg Calcium • 2 gm Fiber

DIABETIC: 1½ Meat • 1 Vegetable • ½ Starch

Fresh Tomato Pizza

If you've never made homemade pizza because it seemed like too much trouble, let me convince you otherwise! This easy-to-use packaged crust sets the stage for a truly scrumptious tomato-y pie so tasty and flavorful, you may never order in again!   ☻   Serves 8

> 1 (11-ounce) can Pillsbury refrigerated crusty French loaf
> 1 (8-ounce) package Philadelphia fat-free cream cheese
> ½ cup Kraft fat-free mayonnaise
> 1½ teaspoons dried basil
> ½ teaspoon dried minced garlic
> 1 teaspoon dried parsley flakes
> 4 cups peeled and sliced fresh tomatoes
> 1 cup chopped onion
> 1 cup chopped fresh mushrooms
> 1½ cups (6 ounces) shredded Kraft reduced-fat mozzarella cheese

Preheat oven to 415 degrees. Spray a 10-by-15-inch rimmed baking sheet with butter-flavored cooking spray. Unroll French loaf and pat into prepared baking sheet. Bake for 6 to 8 minutes or until lightly browned. Meanwhile, in a medium bowl, stir cream cheese with a spoon until soft. Stir in mayonnaise, basil, garlic, and parsley flakes. Spread mixture over partially baked crust. Evenly sprinkle tomatoes, onion, and mushrooms over cream cheese mixture. Sprinkle mozzarella cheese evenly over top. Continue baking for 8 to 10 minutes. Place baking sheet on a wire rack and let set for 5 minutes. Cut into 8 servings.

Each serving equals:

HE: 1½ Protein • 1½ Vegetable • ⅔ Bread •
10 Optional Calories

221 Calories • 5 gm Fat • 16 gm Protein •
28 gm Carbohydrate • 794 mg Sodium •
166 mg Calcium • 2 gm Fiber

DIABETIC: 1½ Meat • 1½ Vegetable •
1 Starch /Carbohydrate

Mediterranean Pizza

When I think of the luscious flavors of the cuisines that border this beautiful sea, I know I can enjoy some of the culinary delights of European travel without leaving my kitchen! This is a spectacular end-of-summer supper that is a great way to use up some of your abundant zucchini harvest. ☻ Serves 8

1 (11-ounce) can Pillsbury refrigerated crusty French loaf
1¾ cups (one 15-ounce can) Hunt's Tomato Sauce
1½ teaspoons dried basil
½ teaspoon dried minced garlic
1 teaspoon dried parsley flakes
1 tablespoon pourable Sugar Twin
2½ cups chopped unpeeled zucchini
¾ cup (3 ounces) crumbled feta cheese
¾ cup (3 ounces) shredded Kraft reduced-fat mozzarella cheese

Preheat oven to 415 degrees. Spray a 10-by-15-inch rimmed baking sheet with olive oil–flavored cooking spray. Unroll French loaf and pat into prepared baking sheet. Bake for 6 to 8 minutes, or until lightly browned. In a small bowl, combine tomato sauce, basil, garlic, parsley flakes, and Sugar Twin. Spread sauce mixture evenly over partially baked crust. Arrange zucchini evenly over sauce. Evenly sprinkle feta and mozzarella cheeses over top. Continue baking for 8 to 10 minutes. Place baking sheet on a wire rack and let set for 5 minutes. Cut into 8 servings.

Each serving equals:

HE: 1½ Vegetable • 1 Bread • 1 Protein •
1 Optional Calorie

173 Calories • 5 gm Fat • 9 gm Protein •
23 gm Carbohydrate • 758 mg Sodium •
135 mg Calcium • 2 gm Fiber

DIABETIC: 1 Vegetable • 1 Starch • 1 Meat

Catch-of-the-Day Fish

When a restaurant waiter regales you with the chef's chosen specials, including a delectable fish dish, it's hard not to be tempted! But if the nearest fresh fish market is miles away, don't despair—just open your freezer, take down a few spices, and wait for the applause! ○ Serves 4

½ cup Kraft fat-free mayonnaise
1 teaspoon dried minced garlic
1 teaspoon lemon juice
1 teaspoon dried parsley flakes
1 teaspoon dried dill weed
16 ounces frozen white fish, thawed, and cut into 4 pieces

In a small bowl, combine mayonnaise, garlic, lemon juice, parsley flakes, and dill weed. Spread about 1 tablespoon mayonnaise mixture over the top of each fish piece. Place fish, mayonnaise-coated side down, in a large skillet sprayed with butter-flavored cooking spray and evenly spread about 1 tablespoon mayonnaise mixture over the prepared side of each fish piece. Cook over medium heat for about 5 minutes on each side or until fish flakes easily.

Each serving equals:

HE: 2 Protein • ¼ Slider

113 Calories • 1 gm Fat • 21 gm Protein •
5 gm Carbohydrate • 353 mg Sodium •
46 mg Calcium • 0 gm Fiber

DIABETIC: 3 Meat

Baked Fish with Corn Salsa

This tangy, crusty fish dish is so moist and full of flavor, you might not believe that something this luscious is also good for you! If you've never been a big fan of fish but you know you should be eating it more often, here's a good way to start. ☾ Serves 4

> 6 tablespoons (1½ ounces) dried fine bread crumbs
> 1 teaspoon dried parsley flakes
> ¼ cup Kraft Fat Free Ranch Dressing
> 16 ounces frozen white fish, thawed, and cut into 4 pieces
> 1 cup frozen whole-kernel corn, thawed
> ½ cup chunky salsa (mild, medium, or hot)

Preheat oven to 350 degrees. Spray an 8-by-8-inch baking dish with butter-flavored cooking spray. In a sealed sandwich bag, combine bread crumbs and parsley flakes. Pour Ranch dressing into a saucer. Coat fish pieces in dressing, then place in sandwich bag, one piece at a time, and shake well to coat fish. Arrange fish pieces in prepared baking dish. Bake for 10 minutes. Meanwhile, in a small bowl, combine corn and salsa. Evenly spoon corn mixture over partially baked fish. Continue baking for 8 to 12 minutes or until fish flakes easily with a fork. Divide into 4 servings.

HINT: Thaw corn by placing in a colander and rinsing under hot water for one minute.

Each serving equals:

HE: 2 Protein • 1 Bread • ¼ Vegetable • ¼ Slider • 5 Optional Calories

---

197 Calories • 1 gm Fat • 24 gm Protein • 23 gm Carbohydrate • 456 mg Sodium • 110 mg Calcium • 2 gm Fiber

---

DIABETIC: 3 Meat • 1½ Starch

Tuna-Stuffed Baked Tomatoes

Stuffing a raw tomato with a scoop of tuna is a classic diner lunch, but I thought I'd transform that American favorite by adding a few delicious ingredients (reduced-fat cheese, fat-free sour cream) and baking up a little magic!   ○   Serves 4

> 4 (medium-sized) fresh tomatoes
> 1 (6-ounce) can white tuna, packed in water, drained and flaked
> 6 tablespoons (1½ ounces) dried fine bread crumbs
> 2 teaspoons dried onion flakes
> ¼ cup Kraft Fat Free Italian Dressing
> ¾ cup (3 ounces) shredded Kraft reduced-fat mozzarella cheese ☆
> ¼ cup Land O Lakes no-fat sour cream

Preheat oven to 400 degrees. Cut a thin slice from top of each tomato. Scoop out center, leaving a ½-inch shell. Place tomatoes cut side down on paper towels to drain. Meanwhile, in a medium bowl, combine tuna, bread crumbs, onion flakes, Italian dressing, and ½ cup mozzarella cheese. Evenly spoon about ½ cup tuna mixture into each tomato shell. Arrange stuffed tomatoes in an 8-by-8-inch baking dish. Sprinkle 1 tablespoon mozzarella cheese over top of each. Bake for 20 to 25 minutes. Place baking dish on a wire rack and let set for 5 minutes. When serving, top each with 1 tablespoon sour cream.

Each serving equals:

HE: 2 Protein • 1 Vegetable • ½ Bread • ¼ Slider • 3 Optional Calories

---

193 Calories • 5 gm Fat • 20 gm Protein • 17 gm Carbohydrate • 568 mg Sodium • 205 mg Calcium • 2 gm Fiber

---

DIABETIC: 2 Meat • 1 Vegetable • 1 Starch/Carbohydrate

Salmon Loaf with Tomato-Dill Sauce

I started with a beloved 1950s dish, the seafood meatloaf enjoyed in homes all over America. But I'm bringing this "golden oldie" into the millennium with a special touch—a dill-flavored tomato sauce to help you live healthy in the new century! ☻ Serves 6

⅔ cup Carnation Nonfat Dry Milk Powder

1¼ cups water

2 teaspoons prepared mustard

1 (14¾-ounce) can pink salmon, boned, skinned, drained, and flaked

¼ cup chopped onion

½ cup finely chopped celery

28 small fat-free saltine crackers, made into crumbs

1 egg or equivalent in egg substitute

2 teaspoons dried dill weed ☆

1 (10¾-ounce) can Healthy Request Tomato Soup

⅓ cup skim milk

1 tablespoon dried onion flakes

Preheat oven to 350 degrees. Spray a 9-by-5-inch loaf pan with butter-flavored cooking spray. In a large bowl, combine dry milk powder, water, and mustard. Add salmon, onion, celery, cracker crumbs, egg, and 1 teaspoon dill weed. Mix well to combine. Let set for 2 to 3 minutes for crackers to absorb moisture. Pat mixture into prepared loaf pan. Bake for 45 to 50 minutes. Place loaf pan on a wire rack while preparing sauce. In a small saucepan, combine tomato soup, skim milk, onion flakes, and remaining 1 teaspoon dill weed. Cook over medium heat for 6 to 8 minutes or until mixture is heated through, stirring occasionally. Cut salmon loaf into 6 pieces. For each serving, place 1 piece of salmon loaf on a plate and spoon a scant ¼ cup sauce over top.

HINT: A self-seal sandwich bag works great for crushing crackers.

Each serving equals:

HE: 2½ Protein • ⅔ Bread • ⅓ Skim Milk • ¼ Vegetable • ¼ Slider • 15 Optional Calories

214 Calories • 6 gm Fat • 18 gm Protein • 22 gm Carbohydrate • 758 mg Sodium • 235 mg Calcium • 1 gm Fiber

DIABETIC: 2½ Meat • 1½ Starch

Salmon-Celery Bake

Here's a pretty dish that takes very little preparation time and would be terrific for an early spring bridal shower or anniversary luncheon. Did you know that in England, people often honor important guests by serving salmon dishes rather than beef?

○ Serves 6

> 1 (14¾-ounce) can pink salmon, boned, skinned,
>   drained and flaked
> 9 tablespoons (2¼ ounces) dried fine bread crumbs
> ¼ cup finely chopped onion
> 1¼ cup finely chopped celery
> 1 (10¾-ounce) can Healthy Request Cream of Celery or
>   Mushroom Soup
> ¼ cup skim milk
> ½ teaspoon lemon pepper
> 1 teaspoon dried parsley flakes

Preheat oven to 350 degrees. Spray an 8-by-8-inch baking dish with butter-flavored cooking spray. In a large bowl, combine salmon, bread crumbs, onion, and celery. Add celery soup, skim milk, lemon pepper, and parsley flakes. Mix well to combine. Let set for 2 to 3 minutes for crackers to absorb moisture. Pat mixture into prepared baking dish. Bake for 45 to 50 minutes. Place baking dish on a wire rack and let set for 5 minutes. Divide into 6 servings.

Each serving equals:

HE: 2⅓ Protein • ½ Bread • ½ Vegetable •
¼ Slider • 11 Optional Calories

209 Calories • 5 gm Fat • 18 gm Protein •
23 gm Carbohydrate • 516 mg Sodium •
201 mg Calcium • 1 gm Fiber

DIABETIC: 2½ Meat • 1 Starch • ½ Vegetable

Spanish Rice with Shrimp

No time to cook, but tired of frozen dinners that just don't have the home-cooked taste you love? Here's a speedy skillet supper that couldn't be simpler to prepare. It's ready in just minutes, and it's brimming over with spicy flavors that your mouth and tummy will cheer!   ☯   Serves 4 (1 cup)

> 1¾ cups (one 15-ounce can) Hunt's Tomato Sauce
> ¾ cup water
> ½ teaspoon Tabasco sauce
> ½ cup frozen peas, thawed
> 1 cup (3 ounces) uncooked instant Minute Rice
> 1 (6-ounce) package frozen shrimp, thawed
> 1 teaspoon dried parsley flakes
> 1 teaspoon chili seasoning

In a large skillet sprayed with olive oil–flavored cooking spray, combine tomato sauce, water, and Tabasco sauce. Bring mixture to a boil. Stir in peas, uncooked rice, shrimp, parsley flakes, and chili seasoning. Lower heat, cover, and simmer for 10 minutes or until rice is tender, stirring occasionally. Remove from heat.

HINT: Canned shrimp, rinsed and drained, may be substituted for
    frozen.

Each serving equals:

HE: 1¾ Vegetable • 1½ Protein • 1 Bread

---

129 Calories • 1 gm Fat • 13 gm Protein •
17 gm Carbohydrate • 782 mg Sodium •
35 mg Calcium • 3 gm Fiber

DIABETIC: 2 Vegetable • 1½ Meat • 1 Starch

Chinese Walnut Chicken Skillet

One of the things I love best about Chinese food is the wonderful variety in texture each dish contains. Here's a dish with that spirit and pizzazz that you can stir up in any handy pan (you don't need a wok, I promise you!).   ☻   Serves 4 (1 cup)

> 8 ounces skinned and boned uncooked chicken breast,
>   cut into 20 pieces
> 1 cup sliced celery
> ½ cup chopped onion
> 2 cups (one 16-ounce can) Healthy Request Chicken Broth
> 1 tablespoon reduced-sodium soy sauce
> 1 teaspoon Oriental seasoning, optional
> 1⅓ cups (4 ounces) uncooked instant Minute Rice
> ¼ cup (1 ounce) chopped walnuts
> 1 cup sliced fresh mushrooms
> 1 cup fresh snow peas

In a large skillet sprayed with butter-flavored cooking spray, sauté chicken, celery, and onion for 6 to 8 minutes or until chicken and vegetables are browned. Add chicken broth, soy sauce, and Oriental seasoning. Mix well to combine. Bring mixture to a boil. Stir in uncooked rice, walnuts, mushrooms, and snow peas. Lower heat and simmer for 10 to 12 minutes, or until rice is tender, stirring occasionally.

Each serving equals:

HE: 1¾ Protein • 1¾ Vegetable • 1 Bread • ½ Fat • 8 Optional Calories

259 Calories • 7 gm Fat • 24 gm Protein • 25 gm Carbohydrate • 602 mg Sodium • 48 mg Calcium • 4 gm Fiber

DIABETIC: 1½ Meat • 1½ Vegetable • 1 Starch • ½ Fat

Diane's Angel Hair Pasta and Chicken

This is a luscious and satisfying way to serve pasta, yet it's delightfully low in calories and fat! Whether you're simply serving dinner to your family, or making your new neighbors feel welcome, this is a splendid choice. ☻ Serves 4 (1 full cup)

> 12 ounces skinned and boned uncooked chicken breasts,
>   cut into 16 pieces
> 2 cups (one 16-ounce can) Healthy Request Chicken Broth
> 1¾ cups (3 ounces) uncooked angel hair pasta
> ½ cup Land O Lakes no-fat sour cream
> 2 tablespoons skim milk
> ¼ cup (¾ ounce) grated Kraft fat-free Parmesan cheese
> 1 teaspoon dried parsley flakes

In a large skillet sprayed with butter-flavored cooking spray, sauté chicken for 5 minutes. Add chicken broth and uncooked angel hair pasta. Mix well to combine. Continue cooking for 10 minutes or until chicken and pasta are tender and most of the liquid is absorbed, stirring occasionally. Stir in sour cream, skim milk, Parmesan cheese, and parsley flakes. Lower heat and simmer for 5 minutes, stirring occasionally.

Each serving equals:

HE: 2½ Protein • 1 Bread • ½ Slider •
1 Optional Calorie

---

226 Calories • 2 gm Fat • 26 gm Protein •
26 gm Carbohydrate • 420 mg Sodium •
57 mg Calcium • 1 gm Fiber

DIABETIC: 2½ Meat • 1½ Starch

Chicken-Broccoli-Pasta Skillet

One-dish meals are a busy cook's best friends, because both the cooking and the cleanup are made extra-easy! Cliff likes to call these recipes "put-all-the-ingredients-in-the-skillet-and-you've-got-dinner!" Aren't I married to a smart man? Oh yes!

● Serves 4 (1¼ cups)

> 2 cups frozen cut broccoli, thawed
> ½ cup chopped onion
> 1½ cups (8 ounces) diced cooked chicken breast
> 1 (10¾-ounce) can Healthy Request Cream of Chicken Soup
> ¼ cup skim milk
> ¼ cup (¾ ounce) grated Kraft fat-free Parmesan cheese
> ⅛ teaspoon black pepper
> ½ cup (one 2.5-ounce jar) sliced mushrooms, drained
> 2 cups hot cooked rotini pasta, rinsed and drained

In a large skillet sprayed with butter-flavored cooking spray, sauté broccoli, onion, and chicken for 10 minutes, stirring occasionally. Stir in chicken soup, skim milk, Parmesan cheese, and black pepper. Add mushrooms and rotini pasta. Mix well to combine. Lower heat and simmer for 10 minutes, stirring occasionally.

HINTS: 1. Thaw broccoli by placing in a colander and rinsing under hot water for one minute.
2. If you don't have leftovers, purchase a chunk of cooked chicken breast from your local deli.
3. 1½ cups uncooked rotini pasta usually cooks to about 2 cups.

Each serving equals:

HE: 2¼ Protein • 1½ Vegetable • 1 Bread • ½ Slider • 11 Optional Calories

268 Calories • 4 gm Fat • 25 gm Protein • 33 gm Carbohydrate • 499 mg Sodium • 60 mg Calcium • 3 gm Fiber

DIABETIC: 2½ Meat • 1½ Starch • 1½ Vegetable

Quick Chicken Fajitas

If your kids are always begging for fast-food fajitas, show them you're just as good a cook as the folks down at Taco Bell! They'll be thrilled to enjoy the flavors they love, made even tastier in this homemade version. ◑ Serves 4 (2 each)

> ½ cup Kraft Fat Free Italian Dressing
> 1 tablespoon lemon juice
> 1 tablespoon lime juice
> 8 ounces skinned and boned uncooked chicken breast,
>   cut into 16 strips
> 1 cup sliced onion
> 1 cup sliced green bell pepper
> 8 (6-inch) flour tortillas
> ½ cup chunky salsa (mild, medium, or hot)
> 2⅔ tablespoons Land O Lakes no-fat sour cream

In a medium bowl, combine Italian dressing, lemon juice, and lime juice. Add chicken pieces. Mix well to coat chicken. In a large skillet, combine undrained chicken mixture, onion, and green pepper. Cook over medium heat for 10 minutes or until chicken and vegetables are tender, stirring often. Meanwhile, warm tortillas in microwave. For each serving, spoon about ¼ cup chicken mixture on a warm tortilla, then top with 1 tablespoon salsa and 1 teaspoon sour cream. Roll up or serve as is.

Each serving equals:

HE: 2 Bread • 1½ Protein • 1¼ Vegetable •
¼ Slider • 6 Optional Calories

285 Calories • 5 gm Fat • 19 gm Protein •
41 gm Carbohydrate • 783 mg Sodium •
88 mg Calcium • 1 gm Fiber

DIABETIC: 2 Starch • 1½ Meat • 1 Vegetable

Chicken Pot Pie Lasagna

Some of my Healthy Exchanges kitchen help used to tease me about coming up with recipes that blended the leftovers of two other creations. I say, why not? I get some of my best ideas that way! This is a particularly inventive (and low-fat) way to get that pot-pie taste in a lasagna casserole. ☻ Serves 6

1 (10 ¾-ounce) can Healthy Request Cream of Chicken Soup
⅔ cup Carnation Nonfat Dry Milk Powder
½ cup water
1 teaspoon dried parsley flakes
1¼ cups shredded carrots
¼ cup finely diced onion
1 cup finely chopped celery
½ cup (one 2.5-ounce jar) sliced mushrooms, drained
3 cups hot cooked mini lasagna noodles or regular noodles,
    rinsed and drained
1 cup (5 ounces) diced cooked chicken breast
1 cup fat-free cottage cheese
¼ cup (¾ ounce) grated Kraft fat-free Parmesan cheese
¾ cup (3 ounces) shredded Kraft reduced-fat mozzarella cheese

Preheat oven to 350 degrees. Spray an 8-by-12-inch baking dish with olive oil–flavored cooking spray. In a medium saucepan sprayed with butter-flavored cooking spray, combine chicken soup, dry milk powder, and water. Stir in parsley flakes, carrots, onion, celery, and mushrooms. Cook over medium heat for about 5 minutes or until mixture is heated through, stirring often. Remove from heat. Arrange half of noodles in prepared baking dish. Sprinkle half of chicken over noodles. Spoon half of sauce mixture over chicken. In a small bowl, combine cottage cheese and Parmesan cheese. Spread cottage cheese mixture evenly over sauce. Repeat layers. Sprinkle mozzarella cheese evenly over top. Bake for 40 to 45 minutes. Place baking dish on a wire rack and let set for 5 minutes. Divide into 6 servings.

HINTS: 1. 2⅔ cups uncooked noodles usually cooks to about 3 cups.
2. If you don't have leftovers, purchase a chunk of cooked chicken breast from your local deli.

Each serving equals:

HE: 2 Protein • 1 Bread • 1 Vegetable •
⅓ Skim Milk • ¼ Slider • 10 Optional Calories

285 Calories • 5 gm Fat • 24 gm Protein •
36 gm Carbohydrate • 632 mg Sodium •
231 mg Calcium • 3 gm Fiber

DIABETIC: 2 Meat • 1½ Starch • 1 Vegetable

Tucson Chicken Skillet

Cliff and I have always enjoyed Southwestern food, and now that our son Tommy, daughter-in-law Angie, and grandbaby Chayanne live in Arizona, we put those sun-kissed flavors on the menu more often and think of those we love who live so many miles away from DeWitt, Iowa.   ☾   Serves 6 (1 full cup)

> 16 ounces skinned and boned uncooked chicken breast,
>   cut into 36 pieces
> 3 cups (15 ounces) diced raw potatoes
> ½ cup chopped onion
> 1 cup chopped red bell pepper
> 1¾ cups (one 15-ounce can) Hunt's Tomato Sauce
> ½ cup water
> 1½ teaspoons dried basil
> ½ teaspoon dried minced garlic
> 1 teaspoon dried parsley flakes
> 2½ cups frozen cut green beans, thawed

In a large skillet sprayed with olive oil–flavored cooking spray, sauté chicken for 5 minutes, or until lightly browned. Add potatoes, onion, and red pepper. Mix well to combine. Continue cooking for 5 minutes, stirring occasionally. Stir in tomato sauce, water, basil, garlic, parsley flakes, and green beans. Lower heat, cover, and simmer for 20 to 25 minutes, or until chicken and potatoes are tender, stirring occasionally.

HINT: Thaw green beans by placing in a colander and rinsing under hot water for one minute.

Each serving equals:

HE: 2½ Vegetable • 2 Protein • ½ Bread

170 Calories • 2 gm Fat • 20 gm Protein •
18 gm Carbohydrate • 523 mg Sodium •
34 mg Calcium • 4 gm Fiber

DIABETIC: 2 Vegetable • 2 Meat • ½ Starch

Country Club Pizza

Suppose you love the ingredients in the traditional club sandwich, but your kids really want pizza for lunch. Why not make everyone happy with this recipe for fun food that's also good for you? It's a great choice for a teen's birthday party! ☻ Serves 8

1 (8-ounce) can Pillsbury Reduced Fat Crescent Rolls
½ cup Kraft fat-free mayonnaise
1 teaspoon lemon juice
1 teaspoon dried basil
2 cups finely shredded lettuce

1½ cups (8 ounces) diced cooked turkey breast
¾ cup (3 ounces) shredded Kraft reduced-fat Cheddar cheese
1 cup chopped fresh tomato
¼ cup Hormel Bacon Bits

Preheat oven to 415 degrees. Spray a rimmed 10-by-15-inch baking sheet with olive oil–flavored cooking spray. Gently pat crescent rolls into pan, being sure to seal perforations. Prick crust with tines of a fork. Bake for 5 to 7 minutes or until lightly browned. Place baking sheet on a wire rack and let set for 10 minutes. In a small bowl, combine mayonnaise, lemon juice, and basil. Spread mixture over cooled crust. Evenly layer lettuce, turkey, Cheddar cheese, and tomato over mayonnaise mixture. Sprinkle bacon bits evenly over top. Cut into 8 servings.

HINTS: 1. Do not use inexpensive rolls, as they don't cover the pan properly.
2. If you don't have leftovers, purchase a chunk of cooked turkey breast from your local deli.

Each serving equals:

HE: 1½ Protein • 1 Bread • ¾ Vegetable • ¼ Slider • 3 Optional Calories

179 Calories • 7 gm Fat • 11 gm Protein • 18 gm Carbohydrate • 963 mg Sodium • 84 mg Calcium • 0 gm Fiber

DIABETIC: 1 Meat • 1 Starch • 1 Vegetable

French Onion Skillet

One of the tastiest soup options on many restaurant menus is French onion soup, that scrumptious concoction topped with melted cheese. I must have had that in mind when I created this fast and fabulous skillet dish that celebrates those flavors in a hearty entrée! ● Serves 4 (1 full cup)

> 8 ounces ground 90% lean turkey or beef
> 3 cups chopped onion
> 1¾ cups (one 14½-ounce can) Swanson Beef Broth
> 1 teaspoon dried parsley flakes
> 1¾ cups (3 ounces) uncooked noodles
> 4 (¾-ounce) slices Kraft reduced-fat Swiss cheese, shredded

In a large skillet sprayed with butter-flavored cooking spray, brown meat and onion. Stir in beef broth and parsley flakes. Bring mixture to a boil. Add uncooked noodles. Mix well to combine. Lower heat, cover, and simmer for 10 minutes or until noodles are tender, stirring occasionally. Stir in shredded Swiss cheese. Continue stirring for 2 to 3 minutes or until cheese melts.

Each serving equals:

HE: 2½ Protein • 1½ Vegetable • 1 Bread •
9 Optional Calories

268 Calories • 8 gm Fat • 21 gm Protein •
29 gm Carbohydrate • 475 mg Sodium •
130 mg Calcium • 2 gm Fiber

DIABETIC: 2½ Meat • 1½ Vegetable • 1 Starch

Chuck Wagon Stew

Don't the words "chuck wagon" just remind of you of old cowboy movies, where those hard-working fellows gathered around the campfire and enjoyed bowls of bubbling hot stew? The Brown Sugar Twin in this recipe recalls those smoky barbecue flavors in a simple and satisfying supper dish. ☺ Serves 4 (1¼ cups)

> 8 ounces ground 90% lean turkey or beef
> ½ cup chopped onion
> 1¾ cups (one 15-ounce can) Hunt's Tomato Sauce
> 2 teaspoons chili seasoning
> 1 tablespoon Brown Sugar Twin
> 1 teaspoon dried parsley flakes
> ⅛ teaspoon black pepper
> 6 ounces (one 8-ounce can) red kidney beans, rinsed and drained
> 2 cups (one 16-ounce can) cut green beans, rinsed and drained
> ⅔ cup (2 ounces) uncooked instant Minute Rice

In a large skillet sprayed with butter-flavored cooking spray, brown meat, and onion. Stir in tomato sauce, chili seasoning, Brown Sugar Twin, parsley flakes, black pepper, and kidney beans. Add green beans and uncooked rice. Mix well to combine. Bring mixture to a boil. Lower heat, cover, and simmer for 10 minutes or until rice is tender, stirring occasionally.

Each serving equals:

HE: 3 Vegetable • 2¼ Protein • ½ Bread • 1 Optional Calorie

193 Calories • 5 gm Fat • 15 gm Protein • 22 gm Carbohydrate • 757 mg Sodium • 36 mg Calcium • 6 gm Fiber

DIABETIC: 3 Vegetable • 2 Meat • 1 Starch

Calico Potluck Beans

Beans, beans, beautiful beans . . . If you've been hoping to get more fiber in your diet but weren't sure how to go about it, here's a great place to start! This protein-rich recipe is filling, flavorful, and just full of kitchen magic. Enjoy! ☻   Serves 6 (1 full cup)

> 8 ounces ground 90% lean turkey or beef
> ½ cup chopped onion
> 10 ounces (one 16-ounce can) red kidney beans, rinsed and
> 　　drained
> 10 ounces (one 16-ounce can) butter beans, rinsed and drained
> 2 cups (one 16-ounce can) cut green beans, rinsed and drained
> 2 cups (one 16-ounce can) cut yellow wax beans,
> 　　rinsed and drained
> 1¾ cups (one 15-ounce can) Hunt's Tomato Sauce
> 2 tablespoons Brown Sugar Twin
> 3 tablespoons Hormel Bacon Bits
> ½ teaspoon dried minced garlic

In a large skillet sprayed with butter-flavored cooking spray, brown meat and onion. Pour meat mixture into a slow cooker container. Stir in kidney beans, butter beans, green beans, and wax beans. Add tomato sauce, Brown Sugar Twin, bacon bits, and garlic. Mix well to combine. Cover and cook on LOW for 6 to 8 hours. Stir well before serving.

Each serving equals:

HE: 2⅔ Protein • 2⅔ Vegetable • 14 Optional Calories

239 Calories • 7 gm Fat • 21 gm Protein •
23 gm Carbohydrate • 947 mg Sodium •
53 mg Calcium • 7 gm Fiber

DIABETIC: 2½ Meat • 2 Vegetable • 1 Starch

Busy Day Cabbage "Rolls"

Stuffed cabbage dishes are found in almost all Eastern European cuisines, but traditional recipes can be very time-consuming to prepare. I kept the taste of those dishes in mind when I stirred up this super-speedy casserole version. ◐ Serves 4

> *8 ounces ground 90% lean turkey or beef*
> *½ cup chopped onion*
> *⅔ cup (2 ounces) uncooked instant Minute Rice*
> *⅛ teaspoon black pepper*
> *3 cups shredded cabbage☆*
> *1 (10¾-ounce) can Healthy Request Tomato Soup*
> *2 tablespoons Brown Sugar Twin*
> *1 cup (one 8-ounce can) Hunt's Tomato Sauce*
> *2 tablespoons white vinegar*
> *1 teaspoon dried parsley flakes*

Preheat oven to 350 degrees. Spray an 8-by-8-inch baking dish with butter-flavored cooking spray. In a large skillet sprayed with butter-flavored cooking spray, brown meat and onion. Stir in uncooked rice and black pepper. Arrange 2 cups cabbage in prepared baking dish. Evenly spoon meat mixture over cabbage. Sprinkle remaining 1 cup cabbage over top. In a medium bowl, combine tomato soup, Brown Sugar Twin, tomato sauce, vinegar, and parsley flakes. Pour soup mixture evenly over cabbage. Cover and bake for 1 hour. Uncover, place baking dish on a wire rack, and let set for 5 minutes. Divide into 4 servings.

Each serving equals:

HE: 2¾ Vegetable • 1½ Protein • ½ Bread • ½ Slider • 7 Optional Calories

198 Calories • 6 gm Fat • 13 gm Protein • 23 gm Carbohydrate • 519 mg Sodium • 41 mg Calcium • 3 gm Fiber

DIABETIC: 2½ Vegetable • 1½ Meat • 1 Starch

Mexican Cabbage and Rice Casserole

I love a shortcut as much as anyone, so I often pick up packages of shredded cabbage for dishes like this tangy one! Of course, shredding your own cabbage burns a few calories, it's true, but most of us don't always have the time or the inclination!   ☻   Serves 4

> 8 ounces ground 90% lean turkey or beef
> ½ cup chopped onion
> 3 cups shredded cabbage
> 1 (10¾-ounce) can Healthy Request Tomato Soup
> ½ cup chunky salsa (mild, medium, or hot)
> 1 tablespoon Brown Sugar Twin
> 1 cup hot cooked rice
> ⅓ cup (1½ ounces) shredded Kraft reduced-fat Cheddar cheese

Preheat oven to 350 degrees. Spray an 8-by-8-inch baking dish with olive oil–flavored cooking spray. In a large skillet sprayed with olive oil–flavored cooking spray, brown meat and onion. Stir in cabbage. Continue cooking for 5 minutes, stirring occasionally. Add tomato soup, salsa, Brown Sugar Twin, and rice. Mix well to combine. Pour mixture into prepared baking dish. Bake for 20 minutes. Sprinkle Cheddar cheese evenly over top. Continue baking for 10 minutes. Place baking dish on a wire rack and let set for 2 to 3 minutes. Divide into 4 servings.

HINT: ⅔ cup uncooked rice usually cooks to about 1 cup.

Each serving equals:

HE: 2 Protein • 2 Vegetable • ½ Bread • ½ Slider • 7 Optional Calories

219 Calories • 7 gm Fat • 15 gm Protein • 24 gm Carbohydrate • 490 mg Sodium • 147 mg Calcium • 2 gm Fiber

DIABETIC: 2 Meat • 2 Vegetable • 1 Starch

Enchilada Casserole

I make it a point to try all the new low-fat and fat-free products that come on the market, so you can imagine how delighted I was to discover a reduced-fat tortilla chip that tasted terrific! Now before you get nervous about eating a "dangerous" snack food, remember that each serving contains only half an ounce. Go for it!   ☺   Serves 6

> 8 ounces ground 90% lean turkey or beef
> ½ cup chopped onion
> ½ cup chopped green bell pepper
> 1 cup (one 8-ounce can) Hunt's Tomato Sauce
> 1 cup Healthy Request tomato juice or any reduced-sodium
>   tomato juice
> 1 tablespoon chili seasoning
> 1 cup (3 ounces) coarsely crushed Dorito's "WOW" Tortilla Chips
> ¾ cup (3 ounces) shredded Kraft reduced-fat Cheddar cheese

Place meat, onion, and green pepper in a plastic colander. Set the colander in a glass pie plate. Cover and microwave on HIGH (100% power) for 5 to 6 minutes or until meat is browned, stirring occasionally. In a large bowl, combine tomato sauce, tomato juice, chili seasoning, and browned meat mixture. Arrange crushed tortilla chips in an 8-by-8-inch baking dish. Layer meat mixture and Cheddar cheese over top. Cover and microwave on HIGH for 6 to 8 minutes, turning dish after 3 minutes. Uncover and let set for 5 minutes. Divide into 6 servings.

HINT: If you love green chili peppers, add a 4-ounce can of drained chopped green chilis when adding tomato juice.

Each serving equals:

HE: 1⅔ Protein • 1⅓ Vegetable • ⅔ Bread

143 Calories • 7 gm Fat • 11 gm Protein •
9 gm Carbohydrate • 453 mg Sodium •
111 mg Calcium • 1 gm Fiber

DIABETIC: 1½ Meat • 1 Vegetable • ½ Starch

Chimichangas

True chimichangas are deep-fried, but I love a challenge—and so I decided to create a Healthy Exchanges version that delivered the flavors without all that fat! You'll be astonished to see how well your oven and some quick shots of cooking spray provide a nicely browned, crusty version that's pretty close to the "real thing."

● Serves 4 (2 each)

> 8 ounces ground 90% lean turkey or beef
> ½ cup chopped onion
> ½ teaspoon dried minced garlic
> 1 cup chunky salsa (mild, medium, or hot) ☆
> 1 teaspoon chili seasoning
> 8 (6-inch) flour tortillas
> ¼ cup Land O Lakes no-fat sour cream

Preheat oven to 475 degrees. Spray a 9-by-13-inch baking dish with olive oil–flavored cooking spray. In a large skillet sprayed with olive oil–flavored cooking spray, brown meat and onion. Stir in garlic, ½ cup salsa, and chili seasoning. Lower heat and simmer for 5 minutes. Spoon about ¼ cup meat mixture into center of each tortilla. Fold 2 sides over filling, then fold ends into center. Place seam side down in prepared baking dish. Lightly spray tops with butter-flavored cooking spray. Bake for 12 to 14 minutes or until golden brown. For each serving, place a chimichanga on a serving plate, then spoon 2 tablespoons salsa and 1 tablespoon sour cream over top.

Each serving equals:

> HE: 2 Bread • 1½ Protein • ¾ Vegetable •
> 15 Optional Calories
>
> ---
>
> 276 Calories • 8 gm Fat • 15 gm Protein •
> 36 gm Carbohydrate • 547 mg Sodium •
> 167 mg Calcium • 2 gm Fiber
>
> ---
>
> DIABETIC: 2 Starch • 1½ Meat • 1 Vegetable

Olé Stuffed Peppers

Remember the kind of stuffed peppers you enjoyed as a child? Well, I bet you'll agree these are better than you ever dreamed this old-fashioned dish could be! You'll smile and cheer when the cheese, ham, and salsa set off tastebud fireworks!   ☻   Serves 4

> 4 (medium-sized) green bell peppers
> 4 eggs or equivalent in egg substitute
> 1 cup skim milk
> 3 tablespoons (¾ ounce) dried fine bread crumbs
> ½ cup (3 ounces) finely diced Dubuque 97% fat-free ham or any
>   extra-lean ham
> ¾ cup (3 ounces) shredded Kraft reduced-fat Cheddar cheese
> 1 cup chunky salsa (mild, medium, or hot)
> ¼ cup Land O Lakes no-fat sour cream

Cut tops off green peppers. Remove seeds and membranes. Place green peppers, cut side up, in an 8-by-8-inch glass baking dish. In a medium bowl, combine eggs and skim milk. Add bread crumbs, ham, and Cheddar cheese. Mix well to combine. Evenly fill green peppers with egg mixture. Cover with waxed paper and microwave on HIGH (100% power) for 10 to 12 minutes or until filling is just set. Place baking dish on a wire rack and let set for 3 minutes. For each serving, place 1 stuffed pepper on a serving plate, spoon ¼ cup salsa over top, and garnish with 1 tablespoon sour cream.

Each serving equals:

HE: 2½ Protein (1 limited) • 1¼ Vegetable •
¼ Skim Milk • ¼ Bread • 15 Optional Calories

204 Calories • 8 gm Fat • 16 gm Protein •
17 gm Carbohydrate • 541 mg Sodium •
197 mg Calcium • 1 gm Fiber

DIABETIC: 2½ Meat • 1 Vegetable • ½ Starch

Cannelloni

You'll feel like a true Italian chef when you fix this spectacular stuffed noodle recipe! It takes a bit more work than just boiling up some pasta and sauce, but oh, the result is definitely worth it. The sauce is so rich, you'll be tempted to lick the baking dish.

☻ Serves 6 (2 each)

> 1¼ cups chopped onion ☆
> 1¾ cups (one 14½-ounce can) stewed tomatoes, undrained
> 1 cup (one 8-ounce can) Hunt's Tomato Sauce
> 1 teaspoon basil
> 1 teaspoon sage
> 2 teaspoons pourable Sugar Twin
> 1 (10-ounce) package frozen spinach, thawed and
>   thoroughly drained
> 3 tablespoons Kraft Fat Free Italian Dressing
> 8 ounces ground 90% lean turkey or beef
> 1 teaspoon dried minced garlic
> ¼ cup (¾ ounce) grated Kraft fat-free Parmesan cheese ☆
> 1 egg, beaten, or equivalent in egg substitute
> 1 teaspoon dried parsley flakes
> 3 tablespoons all-purpose flour
> 1 (10¾-ounce) can Healthy Request Cream of Mushroom Soup
> 12 cooked manicotti noodles, rinsed, drained, and cooled

Preheat oven to 375 degrees. In a medium saucepan sprayed with olive oil–flavored cooking spray, sauté ½ cup onion for 5 minutes or until tender. Add undrained stewed tomatoes, tomato sauce, basil, sage, and Sugar Twin. Mix well to combine. Lower heat and simmer. Meanwhile, in a large skillet sprayed with olive oil–flavored cooking spray, sauté remaining ¾ cup onion and spinach for 10 minutes or until any remaining moisture in spinach has evaporated. Stir in Italian dressing, meat, and garlic. Continue cooking until meat is browned, stirring occasionally. Pour meat mixture into a large bowl. Add 2 tablespoons Parmesan cheese and egg. Mix well to combine. Set aside. Stir parsley flakes and flour into mushroom soup. Spoon about ½ cup tomato sauce in bottom of a 9-by-13-inch baking dish. Using a teaspoon, stuff about ¼ cup meat filling into each noodle. Place stuffed noodles over sauce in baking dish. Spoon soup mixture evenly over noodles. Carefully pour remaining tomato sauce over soup mixture. Evenly sprinkle remaining Parmesan cheese over top. Bake for 25 to 30 minutes. Place baking dish on a wire rack and let set for 5 minutes. Divide into 6 servings.

Each serving equals:

HE: 1⅔ Protein • 2 Vegetable • 1⅓ Bread • ¼ Slider • 12 Optional Calories

262 Calories • 6 gm Fat • 15 gm Protein • 37 gm Carbohydrate • 807 mg Sodium • 153 mg Calcium • 4 gm Fiber

DIABETIC: 2 Protein • 2 Vegetable • 1½ Bread

Zucchini Meatloaf Muffins

If you have trouble getting your family to eat their veggies, this might be a clever way to disguise those good-for-you green things in a muffin-shaped meatloaf! The zucchini helps these bake up deliciously moist. ☺ Serves 6

16 ounces ground 90% lean turkey or beef
½ cup + 1 tablespoon (2¼ ounces) dried fine bread crumbs
¼ cup finely chopped onion
¾ cup shredded unpeeled zucchini
2 teaspoons Italian seasoning ☆
1 cup (one 8-ounce can) Hunt's Tomato Sauce ☆
2 teaspoons pourable Sugar Twin
½ cup + 1 tablespoon (2¼ ounces) shredded Kraft
  reduced-fat mozzarella cheese

Preheat oven to 375 degrees. Spray 6 wells of a muffin pan with olive oil–flavored cooking spray. In a large bowl, combine meat, bread crumbs, onion, zucchini, 1 teaspoon Italian seasoning, and ½ cup tomato sauce. Mix well to combine. Evenly divide meat mixture between prepared muffin cups and make an indentation in the center of each. In a small bowl, combine remaining ½ cup tomato sauce, Sugar Twin, and remaining 1 teaspoon Italian seasoning. Stir in mozzarella cheese. Evenly spoon about 1 tablespoon sauce mixture into the indentation of each muffin. Bake for 30 to 35 minutes. Place muffin pan on a wire rack and let set for 5 minutes.

HINT: Fill unused muffin wells with water. It protects the muffin
  pan and ensures even baking.

Each serving equals:

HE: 2½ Protein • 1 Vegetable • ½ Bread •
1 Optional Calorie

192 Calories • 8 gm Fat • 18 gm Protein •
12 gm Carbohydrate • 487 mg Sodium •
90 mg Calcium • 1 gm Fiber

DIABETIC: 2½ Meat • 1 Vegetable • ½ Starch

Hawaiian Meatloaf

If you're oh-so-ready for a vacation, but your budget and work schedule make it impossible, put on your favorite muumuu or Hawaiian shirt and stir up a little tropical delight tonight! A little Don Ho music will put you in the mood, and this "saucy" meatloaf will send you on a pleasant journey—if only in your dreams!

❂ Serves 6

> 16 ounces ground 90% lean turkey or beef
> 6 tablespoons purchased graham cracker crumbs or
>   2 (2½-inch) graham cracker squares, made into crumbs
> ½ cup chopped green bell pepper
> ¼ cup chopped onion
> 2 tablespoons Brown Sugar Twin
> ½ teaspoon ground ginger
> 1 cup (one 8-ounce can) crushed pineapple, packed in fruit juice,
>   drained and ¼ cup liquid reserved

Preheat oven to 350 degrees. Spray an 8-by-8-inch baking dish with butter-flavored cooking spray. In a large bowl, combine meat, graham cracker crumbs, green pepper, onion, Brown Sugar Twin, ginger, and reserved pineapple juice. Mix well to combine. Pat mixture into prepared baking dish. Bake for 25 minutes. Evenly spoon pineapple over partially baked meatloaf. Continue baking for 15 minutes. Place baking dish on a wire rack and let set for 5 minutes. Cut into 6 servings.

Each serving equals:

HE: 2 Protein • ⅓ Bread • ⅓ Fruit • ¼ Vegetable • 2 Optional Calories

---

158 Calories • 6 gm Fat • 14 gm Protein •
12 gm Carbohydrate • 126 mg Sodium •
22 mg Calcium • 1 gm Fiber

DIABETIC: 2 Meat • 1 Starch/Carbohydrate

Oktoberfest Meatloaf

Experimenting with spices is like an adventure in cooking chemistry for me. I knew what I wanted this dish to taste like, but how could I get that tangy-sweet-spicy flavor I envisioned? It was a job for the Jessica Fletcher of the kitchen! I think I solved the mystery, don't you? ☻ Serves 6

> 1 cup (one 8-ounce can) Hunt's Tomato Sauce
> 2 tablespoons white vinegar
> 1 tablespoon Brown Sugar Twin
> 1 teaspoon prepared mustard
> 1 teaspoon pumpkin pie spice
> 16 ounces ground 90% lean turkey or beef
> ½ cup raisins
> 6 tablespoons (1½ ounces) dried fine bread crumbs

Preheat oven to 350 degrees. Spray a 9-by-5-inch loaf pan with butter-flavored cooking spray. In a medium bowl, combine tomato sauce, vinegar, Brown Sugar Twin, mustard, and pumpkin pie spice. In a large bowl, combine meat, raisins, bread crumbs, and ½ cup tomato sauce mixture. Mix well to combine. Pat mixture into prepared loaf pan. Bake for 20 minutes. Evenly spoon remaining sauce mixture over partially baked meatloaf. Continue baking for 30 minutes. Place pan on a wire rack and let set for 5 minutes. Cut into 6 servings.

Each serving equals:

HE: 2 Protein • ⅔ Fruit • ⅔ Vegetable • ⅓ Bread • 1 Optional Calorie

195 Calories • 7 gm Fat • 15 gm Protein • 18 gm Carbohydrate • 392 mg Sodium • 29 mg Calcium • 1 gm Fiber

DIABETIC: 2 Meat • ½ Fruit • ½ Vegetable • ½ Starch/Carbohydrate

Italian Pepper Steak

Peppers are just packed with vitamin C, so when they're in season, I cook with them and chop them into salads as often as possible. For the meat lovers in your family, here's a *bella* way to have your beef—and still live healthy!   ☻   Serves 6

> *16 ounces lean round steak, cut into 32 thin pieces*
> *2 cups chopped green and/or red bell peppers*
> *1 cup chopped onion*
> *1 (10¾-ounce) can Healthy Request Tomato Soup*
> *¼ cup water*
> *2 teaspoons Italian seasoning*
> *½ teaspoon dried minced garlic*
> *3 cups hot cooked spaghetti, rinsed and drained*

In a large skillet sprayed with olive oil–flavored cooking spray, sauté steak, peppers, and onion for 10 minutes or until tender. Stir in tomato soup, water, Italian seasoning, and garlic. Lower heat and simmer for 10 minutes or until mixture is heated through, stirring occasionally. For each serving, place ½ cup spaghetti on a plate and spoon about ¾ cup beef mixture over top.

HINTS: 1. To make slicing beef easier, freeze 1 hour before slicing.
2. 2½ cups broken uncooked spaghetti usually cooks to about 3 cups.

Each serving equals:

HE: 2 Protein • 1 Bread • 1 Vegetable • ¼ Slider • 10 Optional Calories

249 Calories • 5 gm Fat • 21 gm Protein • 30 gm Carbohydrate • 192 mg Sodium • 22 mg Calcium • 2 gm Fiber

DIABETIC: 2 Meat • 1½ Starch • 1 Vegetable

Creamy Swiss Steak

This is a wonderful meaty supper dish that tastes far more "fattening" than it is! If you love luscious gravy on your steak, I invite you to savor this with the kind of satisfaction that comes from knowing you're enjoying the food you love without taking a chance with your health. ❂ Serves 4

> *3 tablespoons all-purpose flour*
> *1 teaspoon dried parsley flakes*
> *4 (3-ounce) lean minute or cube steaks*
> *1 cup sliced onion*
> *1¾ cups (one 15-ounce can) Hunt's Tomato Sauce*
> *1 (10¾-ounce) can Healthy Request Cream of Mushroom Soup*
> *½ cup (one 2.5-ounce jar) sliced mushrooms, undrained*
> *⅛ teaspoon black pepper*

In a small bowl, combine flour and parsley flakes. Coat steaks on both sides in flour mixture. In a large skillet sprayed with butter-flavored cooking spray, lightly brown steaks for 3 minutes on each side. Sprinkle onion evenly over steaks. In a medium bowl, combine tomato sauce, mushroom soup, undrained mushrooms, black pepper, and any remaining flour mixture. Spoon sauce mixture evenly over top. Lower heat, cover, and simmer for 20 minutes or until steaks are tender. When serving, evenly spoon sauce over steaks.

Each serving equals:

> HE: 2½ Vegetable • 2¼ Protein • ¼ Bread •
> ½ Slider • 1 Optional Calorie
>
> ---
> 289 Calories • 9 gm Fat • 32 gm Protein •
> 20 gm Carbohydrate • 894 mg Sodium •
> 70 mg Calcium • 1 gm Fiber
>
> ---
> DIABETIC: 2½ Vegetable • 2 Meat • ½ Starch

Beef Steak in Mushroom Gravy

The men in my life love meat, so I always used to keep lean minute steaks in my freezer. They're great for busy families because they cook so speedily, and as long as you've got some canned soup and a little flour on hand, healthy, tasty gravy is just "minutes" away! ☻ Serves 4

> 6 tablespoons all-purpose flour
> 1 teaspoon dried onion flakes
> 1 teaspoon dried parsley flakes
> 4 (4-ounce) lean minute or cube steaks
> 1 (10 ¾-ounce) can Healthy Request Cream of Mushroom Soup
> ½ cup (one 2.5-ounce jar) sliced mushrooms, drained
> 1¾ cups (one 14½-ounce can) Swanson Beef Broth

In a small bowl, combine flour, onion flakes, and parsley flakes. Coat steaks on both sides in flour mixture. In a large skillet sprayed with butter-flavored cooking spray, lightly brown steaks for 3 minutes on each side. In a large bowl, combine mushroom soup, mushrooms, beef broth, and any remaining flour mixture. Pour soup mixture evenly over steaks. Bring mixture to a boil. Lower heat, cover, and simmer for 20 to 25 minutes or until steaks are tender. When serving, evenly spoon gravy over steaks.

Each serving equals:

HE: 3 Protein • ½ Bread • ¼ Vegetable • ½ Slider • 10 Optional Calories

---

240 Calories • 8 gm Fat • 24 gm Protein • 18 gm Carbohydrate • 834 mg Sodium • 60 mg Calcium • 1 gm Fiber

---

DIABETIC: 3 Meat • 1 Starch /Carbohydrate

Creamy Baked Steak and Veggies

Most of my recipes serve four to six people, but I know what it's like to cook just for the two of you. Now that all my children have left home, dinner is usually just Cliff and me. He was delighted with this rich baked beef-and-veggies dish. ☺ Serves 2

> 2 (4-ounce) lean minute or cube steaks
> ½ cup chopped onion
> ½ cup chopped green bell peppers
> ½ cup (one 2.5-ounce jar) sliced mushrooms, drained
> 1½ tablespoons all-purpose flour
> ⅓ cup Carnation Nonfat Dry Milk Powder
> ¾ cup water
> ⅛ teaspoon black pepper

Preheat oven to 350 degrees. Spray an 8-by-8-inch baking dish with butter-flavored cooking spray. In a medium skillet sprayed with butter-flavored cooking spray, lightly brown meat for 3 minutes on each side. Place browned meat in prepared baking dish. Evenly sprinkle onion, green pepper, and mushrooms over top. In a covered jar, combine flour, dry milk powder, water, and black pepper. Shake well to blend. Pour flour mixture into the same skillet used to brown meat. Cook over medium heat for 6 to 8 minutes or until mixture thickens, stirring often. Evenly spoon hot sauce mixture over vegetables. Cover and bake for 50 minutes. Uncover and continue baking for 10 minutes. When serving, evenly spoon vegetables and "gravy" over meat pieces.

Each serving equals:

> HE: 3 Protein • ¾ Vegetable • ½ Skim Milk • ¼ Bread
>
> ---
>
> 242 Calories • 6 gm Fat • 30 gm Protein • 17 gm Carbohydrate • 285 mg Sodium • 158 mg Calcium • 2 gm Fiber
>
> ---
>
> DIABETIC: 3 Meat • 1 Vegetable • ½ Skim Milk

Sunshine State Simmered Steaks ❄

You might laugh if you peeked inside my refrigerator and saw the row of jars of spreadable fruit lined up! I think I must have every single flavor in there. I use them in many of my best dessert recipes, but every so often, I spoon some into a main dish, and the result is ravishing!   ☻   Serves 4

3 tablespoons all-purpose flour
1 teaspoon dried parsley flakes
4 (4-ounce) lean minute or cube steaks
1 cup unsweetened orange juice
1 cup (two 2.5-ounce jars) sliced mushrooms, drained
2 tablespoons Heinz Light Harvest Ketchup or any
*   reduced-sodium ketchup*
2 tablespoons orange marmalade spreadable fruit
1 tablespoon dried onion flakes

In a small bowl, combine flour and parsley flakes. Coat steaks on both sides in flour mixture. In a large skillet sprayed with butter-flavored cooking spray, lightly brown steaks for 3 minutes on each side. In a medium bowl, combine orange juice, mushrooms, ketchup, spreadable fruit, onion flakes, and any remaining flour. Spoon mixture evenly over steaks. Lower heat, cover, and simmer for 20 to 25 minutes, or until steaks are tender. When serving, evenly spoon sauce over steaks.

Each serving equals:

HE: 3 Protein • 1 Fruit • ½ Vegetable • ¼ Bread •
8 Optional Calories

---

218 Calories • 6 gm Fat • 23 gm Protein •
18 gm Carbohydrate • 359 mg Sodium •
17 mg Calcium • 1 gm Fiber

DIABETIC: 3 Meat • 1 Fruit • ½ Vegetable

Baked Pork Cutlets with Creamy Veggies

For those meat-and-potatoes men who fear the appearance of healthy food on the dinner table, here's a truly convincing way to win them over for keeps! (Don't tell, but it's also a great way to get them eating their vegetables!)   ☻   Serves 4

2 cups shredded cabbage
2 cups (10 ounces) sliced raw potatoes
1 cup sliced carrots
1 cup chopped onion
1 (10¾-ounce) can Healthy Request Cream of
    Mushroom Soup
⅓ cup Carnation Nonfat Dry Milk Powder
1 cup water
1 teaspoon dried parsley flakes
½ cup (one 2.5-ounce jar) sliced mushrooms, drained
4 (4-ounce) lean pork tenderloins or cutlets

Preheat oven to 375 degrees. Spray an 8-by-8-inch baking dish with butter-flavored cooking spray. In a large bowl, combine cabbage, potatoes, carrots, and onion. Spread vegetable mixture into prepared baking dish. In a medium bowl, combine mushroom soup, dry milk powder, water, and parsley flakes. Stir in mushrooms. Evenly spoon soup mixture over vegetables. In a large skillet sprayed with butter-flavored cooking spray, lightly brown pork for 3 or 4 minutes on each side. Evenly arrange browned pork over soup mixture. Cover and bake for 1 hour. Uncover and continue baking for 15 minutes. For each serving, place a tenderloin on a plate and spoon about one full cup vegetable mixture next to it.

HINT: Don't overbrown pork or it will become tough.

Each serving equals:

HE: 3 Protein • 2¼ Vegetable • ½ Bread •
¼ Skim Milk • ½ Slider • 1 Optional Calorie

258 Calories • 6 gm Fat • 24 gm Protein •
27 gm Carbohydrate • 453 mg Sodium •
177 mg Calcium • 3 gm Fiber

DIABETIC: 3 Meat • 1½ Vegetable • 1 Starch

Spanish Zucchini Pork Skillet

I hope you'll want to sample the sizzle in this spicy dish that features pork tenders! It simmers beautifully on the stove while you're relaxing and watching the news, and it uses handy ingredients you're always likely to have in your pantry. Olé!

○ Serves 6 (1 full cup)

4 (4-ounce) lean pork tenderloins or cutlets, cut into 24 pieces
²⁄₃ cup (2 ounces) uncooked instant Minute Rice
4 cups (two 16-ounce cans) tomatoes, coarsely chopped and
        undrained
¾ cup chopped green bell pepper
¾ cup chopped onion
⅓ cup (1½ ounces) sliced ripe olives
1 tablespoon pourable Sugar Twin
2 cups thinly sliced unpeeled zucchini
1 teaspoon chili seasoning
¼ cup water

In a large skillet sprayed with olive oil–flavored cooking spray, brown meat. Add uncooked rice, undrained tomatoes, green pepper, onion, olives, and Sugar Twin. Mix well to combine. Stir in zucchini, chili seasoning, and water. Lower heat, cover, and simmer for 30 minutes, stirring occasionally.

Each serving equals:

HE: 2½ Vegetable • 2 Protein • ⅓ Bread • ¼ Fat •
1 Optional Calorie

184 Calories • 4 gm Fat • 15 gm Protein •
22 gm Carbohydrate • 341 mg Sodium •
71 mg Calcium • 3 gm Fiber

DIABETIC: 2½ Vegetable • 2 Meat • ½ Starch

Italian Pork Pot

What's lovable about a slow cooker recipe? Simply put, you place all your ingredients in the pot, you turn it on, and you do what you need to do for the next few hours. When you come home, the aroma tells you that supper's ready, and you can be a guest at your own table!   ☉   Serves 4 (1 full cup)

16 ounces lean pork tenderloins or cutlets, cut into 32 pieces
1 (10¾-ounce) can Healthy Request Cream of Mushroom Soup
1¾ cups (one 15-ounce can) Hunt's Tomato Sauce
½ cup chopped onion
1 teaspoon Italian seasoning
1 teaspoon dried parsley flakes
1¾ cups (3 ounces) uncooked noodles

In a slow cooker container, combine pork, mushroom soup, tomato sauce, onion, Italian seasoning, and parsley flakes. Stir in uncooked noodles. Cover and cook on LOW for 6 to 8 hours. Mix well just before serving.

Each serving equals:

HE: 3 Protein • 2 Vegetable • 1 Bread • ½ Slider •
1 Optional Calorie

302 Calories • 6 gm Fat • 31 gm Protein •
31 gm Carbohydrate • 997 mg Sodium •
37 mg Calcium • 2 gm Fiber

DIABETIC: 3 Meat • 2 Vegetable • 1½ Starch

Asparagus Brunch Bake

Instead of a dinner party for your favorite friends, why not invite them over for a cozy end-of-winter brunch that features this dish? I often encourage you to use fresh veggies in my recipes, but this one works better with frozen asparagus.

◐ Serves 6

> 1½ cups (one 12-ounce can) Carnation Evaporated
>   Skim Milk
> 3 tablespoons all-purpose flour
> 1 full cup (6 ounces) diced cooked chicken breast
> ½ cup frozen peas, thawed
> ½ cup (one 2.5-ounce jar) sliced mushrooms, drained
> ¼ cup (one 2-ounce jar) diced pimiento, drained
> ¼ teaspoon lemon pepper
> 1 (10-ounce) package frozen cut asparagus, thawed
> 1 full cup (6 ounces) diced Dubuque 97% fat-free ham or
>   any extra-lean ham
> 6 tablespoons (1½ ounces) dried fine bread crumbs

Preheat oven to 350 degrees. Spray an 8-by-8-inch baking dish with butter-flavored cooking spray. In a covered jar, combine evaporated skim milk and flour. Shake well until blended. Pour mixture into a medium saucepan sprayed with butter-flavored cooking spray. Add chicken, peas, mushrooms, pimiento, and lemon pepper. Cook over medium heat until mixture thickens, stirring often. Remove from heat. Place asparagus in prepared baking dish. Sprinkle ham over asparagus. Evenly spoon warm chicken mixture over ham. Sprinkle bread crumbs evenly over top. Bake for 35 to 40 minutes. Place baking dish on a wire rack and let set for 5 minutes. Divide into 6 servings.

HINT: If you don't have leftovers, purchase a chunk of cooked
    chicken breast from your local deli.

Each serving equals:

HE: 1⅔ Protein • ¾ Vegetable • ⅔ Bread • ½ Skim Milk

203 Calories • 3 gm Fat • 22 gm Protein • 22 gm Carbohydrate • 586 mg Sodium • 194 mg Calcium • 4 gm Fiber

DIABETIC: 2 Meat • 1 Starch • 1 Vegetable • ½ Skim Milk

Ham and Green Beans with Noodles

I choose not to cook with fat-free cheese because I'm not satisfied with its flavor, taste, or "meltability." But oh my goodness, what a wonderful thing happened when they figured out how to make a scrumptious fat-free sour cream! This dish demonstrates how just rich and creamy healthy food can be!   ☺   Serves 4 (1 cup)

1 (10¾-ounce) can Healthy Request Cream of Mushroom Soup
¼ cup Land O Lakes no-fat sour cream
¼ cup (¾ ounce) grated Kraft fat-free Parmesan cheese
2 cups (one 16-ounce can) cut green beans, rinsed and drained
1½ cups (9 ounces) diced Dubuque 97% fat-free ham or any
   extra-lean ham
2 cups hot cooked noodles, rinsed and drained

In a large skillet sprayed with butter-flavored cooking spray, combine mushroom soup, sour cream, and Parmesan cheese. Cook over medium heat for 4 to 5 minutes or until mixture is heated through, stirring occasionally. Add green beans, ham, and noodles. Mix well to combine. Lower heat and simmer for 10 minutes, stirring occasionally.

HINT: 1¾ cups uncooked noodles usually cooks to about 2 cups.

Each serving equals:

HE: 1¾ Protein • 1 Bread • 1 Vegetable • ½ Slider •
16 Optional Calories

245 Calories • 5 gm Fat • 16 gm Protein •
34 gm Carbohydrate • 886 mg Sodium •
77 mg Calcium • 2 gm Fiber

DIABETIC: 2 Meat • 1½ Starch • 1 Vegetable

Boiled Cabbage with Deluxe Ham Sauce

If you love coleslaw but don't know whether you'll like boiled cabbage, give this creamy, cheesy dish a chance to win your heart (and tummy!). The ham and Swiss cheese sauce is downright irresistible!

❍ Serves 4

> 6 cups coarsely chopped cabbage
> 3 cups hot water
> 1 full cup (6 ounces) diced Dubuque 97% fat-free ham or any
>   extra-lean ham
> 1 cup shredded carrots
> 1½ cups (one 12-ounce can) Carnation Evaporated Skim Milk
> 3 tablespoons all-purpose flour
> 4 (¾-ounce) slices Kraft reduced-fat Swiss cheese, shredded
> ⅛ teaspoon black pepper

In a large saucepan, combine cabbage and water. Bring mixture to a boil. Lower heat and cook for 15 minutes or until cabbage is just tender. Meanwhile, in a large skillet sprayed with butter-flavored cooking spray, sauté ham and carrots for 5 minutes. In a covered jar, combine evaporated skim milk and flour. Shake well to blend. Add milk mixture to ham mixture. Stir in Swiss cheese and black pepper. Lower heat and simmer for 10 minutes or until mixture thickens and cheese melts, stirring often. Drain cabbage. For each serving, place about 1 full cup of cabbage on a plate and spoon about ⅔ cup ham sauce over top.

Each serving equals:

HE: 3½ Vegetable • 2 Protein • ¾ Skim Milk • ¼ Bread

207 Calories • 3 gm Fat • 22 gm Protein •
23 gm Carbohydrate • 548 mg Sodium •
524 mg Calcium • 2 gm Fiber

DIABETIC: 2½ Vegetable • 2 Meat • 1 Skim Milk

Calico Potato and Ham Bake

Be prepared to hear, "When will dinner be ready?" for nearly an hour once the delectable aroma of this cheesy dish begins floating out of your kitchen and around your house! Just smile and say, "Good things are worth waiting for!" ☻ Serves 6

> 1 cup frozen whole-kernel corn, thawed
> 2 cups frozen cut broccoli, thawed
> 3 cups (10 ounces) frozen loose-packed shredded potatoes
> 1½ cups (9 ounces) diced Dubuque 97% fat-free ham or any
>   extra-lean ham
> ¾ cup (3 ounces) shredded Kraft reduced-fat Cheddar cheese
> 1 (10¾-ounce) can Healthy Request Cream of Mushroom Soup
> 1 teaspoon dried onion flakes
> ⅛ teaspoon black pepper

Preheat oven to 350 degrees. Spray an 8-by-12-inch baking dish with butter-flavored cooking spray. In a large bowl, combine corn, broccoli, potatoes, and ham. Stir in Cheddar cheese. Add mushroom soup, onion flakes, and black pepper. Mix well to combine. Spread mixture into prepared baking dish. Bake for 45 to 50 minutes. Place baking dish on a wire rack and let set for 5 minutes. Divide into 6 servings.

HINTS: 1. Thaw corn and broccoli by placing in a colander and rinsing under hot water for one minute.
2. Mr. Dell's frozen shredded potatoes are a good choice, or raw shredded potatoes may be used in place of frozen potatoes.

Each serving equals:

HE: 1⅔ Protein • ⅔ Bread • ⅔ Vegetable • ¼ Slider • 7 Optional Calories

181 Calories • 5 gm Fat • 13 gm Protein • 21 gm Carbohydrate • 633 mg Sodium • 150 mg Calcium • 3 gm Fiber

DIABETIC: 1½ Meat • 1 Starch • ½ Vegetable

Dixie Dandy Bake

I had fun naming this recipe—can't you tell? But what a dandy treat it is, filled with so much fruity pleasure your mouth may start to water as you read the list of ingredients. This would be wonderful on a holiday buffet, but it's great anytime! ☻ Serves 6

> 1 cup unsweetened applesauce
> 1 cup (one 8-ounce can) pineapple tidbits, packed in fruit juice,
>   drained, and 2 tablespoons liquid reserved
> 1½ cups (9 ounces) diced Dubuque 97% fat-free ham or any
>   extra-lean ham
> 4½ cups (24 ounces) peeled and sliced cooked sweet potatoes
> 2 tablespoons apricot spreadable fruit
> 1 teaspoon prepared mustard

Preheat oven to 400 degrees. Spray an 8-by-8-inch baking dish with butter-flavored cooking spray. In a large bowl, combine applesauce, pineapple, ham, and sweet potatoes. Evenly spread mixture into prepared baking dish. In a small bowl, combine apricot spreadable fruit, reserved pineapple liquid, and mustard. Drizzle mixture evenly over sweet potato mixture. Bake for 35 to 40 minutes. Place baking dish on a wire rack and let set for 5 minutes. Divide into 6 servings.

HINT: If you can't find tidbits, use chunk pineapple and coarsely chop.

Each serving equals:

HE: 1 Bread • 1 Protein • 1 Fruit

198 Calories • 2 gm Fat • 9 gm Protein •
36 gm Carbohydrate • 432 mg Sodium •
33 mg Calcium • 4 gm Fiber

DIABETIC: 1½ Starch • 1 Meat • 1 Fruit

Chef's Salad Sandwich Wedges

It's a salad! It's a sandwich! Why, it's two, two, two-in-one! I thought it might be fun to savor the flavors of a chef's salad piled high on a wonderfully flaky crust. This looks absolutely beautiful, and it tastes even better than it looks. ☻ Serves 8 (3 each)

1 (8-ounce) can Pillsbury Reduced Fat Crescent Rolls
1 (8-ounce) package Philadelphia fat-free cream cheese
¼ cup Kraft fat-free mayonnaise
¼ cup Kraft Fat Free Ranch Dressing
2½ cups finely shredded lettuce
¼ cup sliced green onion
½ cup shredded carrots
¾ cup finely chopped fresh tomatoes
1 cup (6 ounces) diced Dubuque 97% fat-free ham or any
    extra-lean ham
¾ cup (3 ounces) shredded Kraft reduced-fat Cheddar cheese
2 hard-boiled eggs, diced
½ cup Kraft Fat Free Catalina Dressing

Preheat oven to 415 degrees. Spray a rimmed 10-by-15 inch baking sheet with butter-flavored cooking spray. Gently pat crescent rolls into pan, being sure to seal perforations. Prick crust with tines of a fork. Bake for 8 to 10 minutes or until lightly browned. Place baking sheet on a wire rack and let set for 10 minutes. Meanwhile, in a medium bowl, stir cream cheese with a spoon until soft. Add mayonnaise and Ranch dressing. Mix well to combine. Spread mixture evenly over cooled crust. In a medium bowl, combine lettuce, green onion, and carrots. Sprinkle lettuce mixture evenly over cream cheese mixture. Evenly sprinkle tomatoes, ham, Cheddar cheese, and eggs over lettuce mixture. Drizzle Catalina dressing evenly over top. Cut into 24 pieces.

HINTS: 1. Do not use inexpensive rolls, as they don't cover the pan properly.

2. If you want the look and feel of eggs without the cholesterol, toss out the yolks and dice the whites.

Each serving equals:

HE: 1¾ Protein (¼ limited) • 1 Bread • 1 Vegetable • ½ Slider • 3 Optional Calories

237 Calories • 9 gm Fat • 15 gm Protein • 24 gm Carbohydrate • 983 mg Sodium • 101 mg Calcium • 1 gm Fiber

DIABETIC: 2 Meat • 1½ Starch • 1 Vegetable

Reuben Biscuit Cups

It's one of America's most beloved deli sandwiches, but instead of heading to the store, you can serve up your own version of this favorite! Kids just love gobbling these down, and they reheat beautifully in a microwave. ☻ Serves 5 (2 each)

1 (7.5-ounce) can Pillsbury refrigerated buttermilk biscuits
2 tablespoons Kraft Fat Free Thousand Island Dressing
2 tablespoons Kraft fat-free mayonnaise
¼ cup chopped onion
2 (2.5-ounce) packages Carl Buddig 90% lean corned beef, shredded
1 cup (one 8-ounce can) sauerkraut, well drained
5 (¾-ounce) slices Kraft reduced-fat Swiss cheese, shredded

Preheat oven to 400 degrees. Separate biscuits and place each biscuit in an ungreased muffin cup, pressing dough up sides to edge of cup. In a large bowl, combine Thousand Island dressing, mayonnaise, and onion. Add corned beef, sauerkraut, and Swiss cheese. Mix well to combine. Evenly spoon mixture into biscuit cups. Bake for 10 to 15 minutes or until filling is bubbly and biscuits are browned. Place muffin pan on a wire rack and let set for 5 minutes.

HINT: Fill unused muffin wells with water. It protects the muffin pan and ensures even baking.

Each serving equals:

HE: 2 Protein • 1½ Bread • ½ Vegetable • 14 Optional Calories

200 Calories • 4 gm Fat • 15 gm Protein • 26 gm Carbohydrate • 907 mg Sodium • 220 mg Calcium • 4 gm Fiber

DIABETIC: 1½ Meat • 1½ Starch • ½ Vegetable

Corned Beef Skillet Sandwiches

I've served thousands of Healthy JO's, my own version of Sloppy Joes, in my café over the years, but that's not the only tasty meat combo to spoon between two halves of a bun! This corned beef concoction makes for a delectable surprise. ☻ Serves 4

> 2 (2.5-ounce) packages Carl Buddig 90% lean corned beef, shredded
> ¼ cup finely chopped onion
> 1¾ cups (one 14½-ounce can) stewed tomatoes, coarsely chopped and undrained
> 1 teaspoon prepared mustard
> ¾ cup (3 ounces) shredded Kraft reduced-fat Cheddar cheese
> 4 reduced-calorie hamburger buns

In a large skillet sprayed with butter-flavored cooking spray, sauté corned beef and onion for 5 minutes. Stir in undrained tomatoes and mustard. Lower heat and simmer for 15 minutes or until most of the liquid has evaporated, stirring occasionally. Add Cheddar cheese. Mix well to combine. Continue simmering for 5 minutes or until cheese melts, stirring occasionally. For each sandwich, spoon about ⅓ cup mixture between a bun.

Each serving equals:

HE: 2¼ Protein • 1 Bread • 1 Vegetable

211 Calories • 7 gm Fat • 15 gm Protein •
22 gm Carbohydrate • 944 mg Sodium •
200 mg Calcium • 2 gm Fiber

DIABETIC: 2 Meat • 1 Starch • 1 Vegetable

Corned Beef and Cabbage Casserole

You don't have to wait for St. Patrick's Day to eat this Irish standby! You can feel confident enjoying my Healthy Exchanges version that banishes most of the fat but still delivers a great big *shillelagh* of flavor!   ☺   Serves 8

> 6 cups (20 ounces) frozen loose-packed
>   shredded potatoes
> 1 cup chopped onion
> 2 cups thinly sliced carrots
> 3 cups shredded cabbage
> 4 (2.5-ounce) packages Carl Buddig 90% lean
>   corned beef, shredded
> 1 (10¾-ounce) can Healthy Request Cream of Celery
>   or Mushroom Soup
> ½ cup skim milk
> 8 (¾-ounce) slices Kraft reduced-fat
>   Swiss cheese

Preheat oven to 350 degrees. Spray a 9-by-13-inch baking dish with butter-flavored cooking spray. Evenly arrange potatoes in prepared baking dish. Layer onion, carrots, cabbage, and corned beef over top. In a medium bowl, combine celery soup and skim milk. Spoon mixture evenly over corned beef mixture. Cover and bake for 60 minutes. Uncover and evenly arrange Swiss cheese slices over top. Continue baking for 15 minutes or until vegetables are tender. Place baking dish on a wire rack and let set for 5 minutes. Cut into 8 servings.

HINT: Mr. Dell's frozen shredded potatoes are a good choice, or raw shredded potatoes may be used in place of frozen potatoes.

Each serving equals:

HE: 2 Protein • 1½ Vegetable • ½ Bread • ¼ Slider • 6 Optional Calories

212 Calories • 8 gm Fat • 13 gm Protein • 22 gm Carbohydrate • 894 mg Sodium • 67 mg Calcium • 3 gm Fiber

DIABETIC: 2 Meat • 1½ Vegetable • 1 Starch

Desserts

Chocolate Almond Banana Treats

It was your favorite when you were little, and chocolate pudding still has the power to make you smile on even the toughest days. Here's a more grown-up version of that kiddie treat, and this is comfort food that can really make you feel better!

☺ Serves 4

> 1 (4-serving) package JELL-O sugar-free instant chocolate pudding mix
> ⅔ cup Carnation Nonfat Dry Milk Powder
> 1½ cups water
> ½ cup Cool Whip Free
> 1 teaspoon almond extract
> 2 cups (2 medium) diced bananas
> 2 tablespoons (½ ounce) slivered almonds

In a large bowl, combine dry pudding mix, dry milk powder, and water. Mix well using a wire whisk. Blend in Cool Whip Free and almond extract. Add bananas. Mix gently to combine. Evenly spoon mixture into 4 dessert dishes. Top each with 1½ teaspoons almonds. Refrigerate for at least 10 minutes.

HINT: To prevent bananas from turning brown, mix with 1 teaspoon lemon juice or sprinkle with Fruit Fresh.

Each serving equals:

HE: 1 Fruit • ½ Skim Milk • ¼ Fat • ½ Slider •
12 Optional Calories

---

183 Calories • 3 gm Fat • 6 gm Protein •
33 gm Carbohydrate • 173 mg Sodium •
153 mg Calcium • 2 gm Fiber

DIABETIC: 1 Fruit • ½ Skim Milk •
½ Starch/Carbohydrate • ½ Fat

Caribbean Tapioca Fruit Pudding

This is such a pretty color, you'll feel soothed and satisfied even before you take a bite! All these tropical flavors will make you feel as if you've just returned from a restful cruise.

❍ Serves 8

> 1 (4-serving) package JELL-O sugar-free vanilla
>   cook-and-serve pudding mix
> 3 tablespoons Quick Cooking Minute Tapioca
> 1 (4-serving) package JELL-O sugar-free orange gelatin
> 1 cup (one 8-ounce can) crushed pineapple,
>   packed in fruit juice, undrained
> 1½ cups water
> 1 teaspoon coconut extract
> 1 teaspoon rum extract
> 1 cup (one 11-ounce can) mandarin oranges,
>   rinsed and drained
> ¾ cup Dannon plain fat-free yogurt
> ⅓ cup Carnation Nonfat Dry Milk Powder
> 1 cup Cool Whip Free
> 1 tablespoon + 1 teaspoon flaked coconut

In a large saucepan, combine dry pudding mix, dry tapioca, and dry gelatin. Add undrained pineapple and water. Mix well to combine. Let set for 5 minutes. Cook over medium heat until mixture thickens and starts to boil, stirring often. Remove from heat. Add coconut and rum extracts. Mix well to combine. Place saucepan on a wire rack. Stir in mandarin oranges. Place saucepan on a wire rack and allow to cool for 30 minutes, stirring occasionally. In a large bowl, combine yogurt and dry milk powder. Blend in Cool Whip Free. Add cooled tapioca mixture to yogurt mixture. Mix gently to combine. Evenly spoon mixture into 8 dessert dishes and top each with ½ teaspoon coconut. Refrigerate for at least 30 minutes.

Each serving equals:

HE: ½ Fruit • ¼ Skim Milk • ½ Slider •
4 Optional Calories

84 Calories • 0 gm Fat • 3 gm Protein •
18 gm Carbohydrate • 232 mg Sodium •
43 mg Calcium • 0 gm Fiber

DIABETIC: ½ Fruit • ½ Starch/Carbohydrate

Mexican Mocha Cappuccino Rice Pudding

You just can't have too many rice pudding recipes—every grandma knows that! Especially when your husband and your grandkids love it. I'm not the coffee-flavor fan in our family, but I made sure to try this out on people who are mocha-mad—and they adored it!

◗ Serves 4

1 (4-serving) package JELL-O sugar-free instant chocolate pudding mix

⅔ cup Carnation Nonfat Dry Milk Powder

1 teaspoon dry coffee crystals

½ teaspoon ground cinnamon

1¼ cups water

¼ cup Cool Whip Free

1 teaspoon vanilla extract

1½ cups cold cooked rice

½ cup raisins

In a large bowl, combine dry pudding mix, dry milk powder, coffee crystals, cinnamon, and water. Mix well using a wire whisk. Blend in Cool Whip Free and vanilla extract. Add rice and raisins. Mix gently to combine. Evenly spoon mixture into 4 dessert dishes. Cover and refrigerate for at least 15 minutes.

HINTS: 1. 1 cup uncooked rice usually cooks to about 1½ cups.
2. To plump up raisins without "cooking," place in a glass measuring cup and microwave on HIGH for 20 seconds.

Each serving equals:

HE: 1 Fruit • ¾ Bread • ½ Skim Milk • ¼ Slider • 17 Optional Calories

168 Calories • 0 gm Fat • 6 gm Protein • 36 gm Carbohydrate • 401 mg Sodium • 156 mg Calcium • 1 gm Fiber

DIABETIC: 1 Fruit • 1 Starch • ½ Skim Milk

Baked Pumpkin Pecan Pudding

I promise you, the calorie count for this scrumptious dessert is absolutely correct! Because you start with pumpkin instead of pudding mix, and because you use egg whites, which have almost no calories, you're ahead from the start. None of that would matter, of course, if it didn't taste downright spectacular—which it DOES.

● Serves 8

> 2 cups (one 15-ounce can) pumpkin
> 2 tablespoons Brown Sugar Twin
> 1½ teaspoons pumpkin pie spice
> ¼ cup (1 ounce) chopped pecans
> 6 egg whites
> ½ cup pourable Sugar Twin
> 1 teaspoon vanilla extract
> 1 cup water

Preheat oven to 300 degrees. In a large bowl, combine pumpkin, Brown Sugar Twin, pumpkin pie spice, and pecans. In a medium bowl, beat egg whites with an electric mixer until soft peaks form. Add Sugar Twin and vanilla extract. Continue beating until stiff peaks form. Using a rubber spatula, carefully fold egg mixture into pumpkin mixture. Spoon mixture into 8 (6-ounce) custard cups. Place cups in a 9-by-13-inch cake pan. Carefully pour water into bottom of pan. Bake for 1 hour. Place custard cups on a wire rack and let set for at least 5 minutes.

Each serving equals:

> HE: ½ Fat • ½ Vegetable • ¼ Protein • 7 Optional Calories
>
> 54 Calories • 2 gm Fat • 3 gm Protein • 6 gm Carbohydrate • 44 mg Sodium • 19 mg Calcium • 2 gm Fiber
>
> DIABETIC: ½ Fat • ½ Starch/Carbohydrate

Apple Noodle Pudding

Noodles for dessert? It may sound a bit unusual, but it's also absolutely delicious! The creamy sauce and fragrant spiced apples will warm you heart and soul. ☻ Serves 6

> 1 (4-serving) package JELL-O sugar-free vanilla cook-and-serve
>   pudding mix
> ⅔ cup Carnation Nonfat Dry Milk Powder
> 1½ cups water
> 1 teaspoon apple pie spice
> 2 cups hot cooked noodles, rinsed and drained
> ¼ cup (1 ounce) chopped walnuts
> 1½ cups (3 small) peeled and diced cooking apples
> 6 tablespoons raisins

Preheat oven to 350 degrees. Spray an 8-by-8-inch baking dish with butter-flavored cooking spray. In a large saucepan, combine dry pudding mix, dry milk powder, and water. Cook over medium heat until mixture thickens and starts to boil, stirring constantly. Remove from heat. Stir in apple pie spice and noodles. Add walnuts, apples, and raisins. Mix well to combine. Spread mixture into prepared baking dish. Bake for 45 to 50 minutes. Place baking dish on a wire rack and let set for 5 minutes. Divide into 6 servings.

HINT: 1¾ cups uncooked noodles usually cooks to about 2 cups.

Each serving equals:

HE: 1 Fruit • ⅔ Bread • ⅓ Skim Milk • ⅓ Fat •
¼ Slider • 3 Optional Calories

---

188 Calories • 4 gm Fat • 6 gm Protein •
32 gm Carbohydrate • 123 mg Sodium •
109 mg Calcium • 2 gm Fiber

DIABETIC: 1 Fruit • 1 Starch/Carbohydrate • ½ Fat

Strawberry Churrios

This Mexican-inspired dessert is wonderfully sweet, so as soon as the berries are RED and RIPE, put this dish on the menu immediately! ☻ Serves 8

> 1 Pillsbury refrigerated unbaked 9-inch piecrust
> ½ cup pourable Sugar Twin ☆
> 1 teaspoon ground cinnamon
> 6 cups sliced fresh strawberries ☆
> 2 tablespoons water
> ½ cup Cool Whip Lite

Preheat oven to 350 degrees. Place piecrust on a large piece of waxed paper and cover with another piece of waxed paper. Roll crust 1 inch larger than original shape. In a small bowl, combine 2 tablespoons Sugar Twin and cinnamon. Evenly sprinkle mixture over piecrust. Cut crust into 32 pie-shaped wedges. Place wedges on a large cookie sheet. Bake for 6 to 8 minutes or until slightly crisp. Place cookie sheet on a wire rack and allow to cool. Meanwhile, in a blender container, combine 2 cups strawberries, water, and remaining 6 tablespoons Sugar Twin. Cover and process on HIGH for 15 seconds. Pour mixture into a large bowl. Stir remaining strawberries into mixture. For each serving, place 4 pie wedges in a dessert bowl, spoon about ⅔ cup strawberry mixture over pie wedges, and top each with 1 tablespoon Cool Whip Lite.

Each serving equals:

HE: ¾ Fruit • ½ Bread • ¾ Slider •
6 Optional Calories

164 Calories • 8 gm Fat • 1 gm Protein •
22 gm Carbohydrate • 101 mg Sodium •
18 mg Calcium • 2 gm Fiber

DIABETIC: 1 Fruit • 1 Fat • ½ Starch

Becky's Peach Strawberry Shortcake

My daughter Becky gave me a new grandbaby to love when she and her husband John recently had a little boy they named Spencer. I was so happy, I immediately stirred up a dessert that includes both her favorites and mine. Cliff and I couldn't be there for the birth, but we celebrated in our own way with a special dessert!

○ Serves 4

> 1 cup (2 medium-sized) peeled and sliced peaches
>
> 1/4 cup water
>
> 6 tablespoons pourable Sugar Twin☆
>
> 2 cups sliced fresh strawberries
>
> 3/4 cup Bisquick Reduced Fat Baking Mix
>
> 1/3 cup Carnation Nonfat Dry Milk Powder
>
> 1 tablespoon (1/4 ounce) chopped pecans
>
> 2 tablespoons Land O Lakes no-fat sour cream
>
> 1/4 cup Cool Whip Lite

Preheat oven to 400 degrees. Spray a baking sheet with butter-flavored cooking spray. In a blender container, combine peaches and water. Cover and process on BLEND for 15 seconds. In a medium bowl, combine peach mixture, 1/4 cup Sugar Twin, and strawberries. Refrigerate until ready to serve. In a large bowl, combine baking mix, dry milk powder, pecans, and remaining 2 tablespoons Sugar Twin. Add remaining 1/2 cup peach mixture and sour cream. Mix well to combine. Drop batter by tablespoon onto prepared baking sheet to form 4 shortcakes. Bake for 8 to 12 minutes or until golden brown. Place baking sheet on a wire rack and let set for at least 5 minutes. For each serving, place 1 shortcake in a dessert dish, spoon about 1/2 cup sauce over top, and garnish with 1 tablespoon Cool Whip Lite.

Each serving equals:

HE: 1 Bread • 1 Fruit • ¼ Skim Milk • ¼ Fat •
¼ Slider • 6 Optional Calories

---

179 Calories • 3 gm Fat • 4 gm Protein •
34 gm Carbohydrate • 360 mg Sodium •
122 mg Calcium • 2 gm Fiber

DIABETIC: 1 Starch • 1 Fruit • ½ Fat

Fruit Cocktail Crumble

This dish is what I'd call a "truckstop delight"—the kind of old-fashioned, down-home, sweet-and-crunchy dessert that appears on so many buffets here in the Midwest. It's easy, cozy, happy food!

Serves 6

9 (2½-inch) graham cracker squares
1 (4-serving) package JELL-O sugar-free vanilla cook-and-serve pudding mix
2 cups (one 16-ounce can) fruit cocktail, packed in fruit juice, undrained
¾ cup water
½ teaspoon ground cinnamon
2 tablespoons pourable Sugar Twin

Preheat oven to 350 degrees. Spray an 8-by-8-inch baking dish with butter-flavored cooking spray. Break graham crackers into large chunks. Evenly sprinkle chunks into prepared baking dish. In a medium saucepan, combine dry pudding mix, undrained fruit cocktail, and water. Cook over medium heat until mixture thickens and starts to boil, stirring often. Pour hot mixture over graham crackers. In a small bowl, combine cinnamon and Sugar Twin. Evenly sprinkle topping mixture over fruit cocktail mixture. Bake for 25 to 30 minutes. Place baking dish on a wire rack and let set for at least 10 minutes. Divide into 6 servings.

HINT: Good served cold with Cool Whip Lite or warm with Wells' Blue Bunny sugar- and fat-free ice cream or any sugar- and fat-free ice cream, but don't forget to count the few additional calories.

Each serving equals:

HE: ⅔ Fruit • ½ Bread • 15 Optional Calories

97 Calories • 1 gm Fat • 1 gm Protein • 21 gm Carbohydrate • 86 mg Sodium • 10 mg Calcium • 1 gm Fiber

DIABETIC: 1 Fruit • ½ Starch

Peach Pecan Cobbler

Okay, maybe your grandma never made peach cobbler for you. That's no reason to live your whole life without it! I've come to the rescue with a simple, tasty version that is utterly delightful. Fresh peaches taste like they're full of sunny sweetness! ☻ Serves 6

1 (4-serving) package JELL-O
  sugar-free vanilla cook-
  and-serve pudding mix
1 (4-serving) package JELL-O
  sugar-free lemon gelatin
1½ cups water
3 cups (6 medium) fresh peeled
  and sliced peaches

½ teaspoon ground nutmeg
3 tablespoons (¾ ounce)
  chopped pecans
1 (7.5-ounce) can Pillsbury
  refrigerated biscuits
¼ cup Cary's Sugar Free
  Maple Syrup

Preheat oven to 375 degrees. Spray an 8-by-8-inch baking dish with butter-flavored cooking spray. In a medium saucepan, combine dry pudding mix, dry gelatin, and water. Add peaches. Mix well to combine. Cook over medium heat until mixture thickens and starts to boil, stirring often. Remove from heat. Stir in nutmeg. Pour mixture into prepared baking dish. Evenly sprinkle pecans over top of peach mixture. Separate biscuits and cut each into 4 pieces. Evenly drop biscuit pieces over pecans. Drizzle maple syrup over top. Bake for 30 minutes. Place baking dish on a wire rack and let set for 5 minutes. Divide into 6 servings.

Each serving equals:

HE: 1¼ Bread • 1 Fruit • ½ Fat • ¼ Slider •
7 Optional Calories

192 Calories • 4 gm Fat • 4 gm Protein •
35 gm Carbohydrate • 439 mg Sodium •
7 mg Calcium • 4 gm Fiber

DIABETIC: 1½ Starch/Carbohydrate • 1 Fruit • ½ Fat

Aloha Fruit Dessert

This was a big hit with Zach and Josh, my two grandsons who often come to visit me in DeWitt. They loved its creamy, fruity goodness, and sweetly asked for "More, please!"

⊘ Serves 8

> 12 (2½-inch) graham cracker squares ☆
> 1 (4-serving) package JELL-O sugar-free vanilla cook-and-serve pudding mix
> 1 (4-serving) package JELL-O sugar-free orange gelatin
> 1 cup (one 8-ounce can) crushed pineapple, packed in fruit juice, undrained
> ¾ cup water
> 1 cup (one 11-ounce can) mandarin oranges, rinsed and drained
> 2 cups (2 medium) diced bananas
> 1 cup Cool Whip Free
> 1 teaspoon coconut extract
> 2 tablespoons (½ ounce) chopped pecans
> 2 tablespoons flaked coconut

Arrange 9 graham crackers in a 9-by-9-inch cake pan. In a medium saucepan, combine dry pudding mix, dry gelatin, undrained pineapple, and water. Cook over medium heat until mixture thickens and starts to boil, stirring often. Remove from heat. Stir in mandarin oranges and bananas. Carefully spoon hot mixture over graham crackers. Refrigerate until firm, about 2 hours. In a medium bowl, combine Cool Whip Free and coconut extract. Spread topping mixture evenly over fruit filling. Finely crush remaining 3 graham crackers. In a medium bowl, combine graham cracker crumbs, pecans, and coconut. Evenly sprinkle crumb mixture over top. Refrigerate for at least 15 minutes. Cut into 8 servings.

HINT: A self-seal sandwich bag works great for crushing graham crackers.

Each serving equals:

HE: 1 Fruit • ½ Bread • ¼ Fat • ¼ Slider •
14 Optional Calories

---

138 Calories • 2 gm Fat • 2 gm Protein •
28 gm Carbohydrate • 129 mg Sodium •
11 mg Calcium • 1 gm Fiber

DIABETIC: 1 Fruit • 1 Starch

Apricot Cobble-Up

Instead of piling the crumb topping on the top, I've secretly hidden it on the bottom of this tasty baked dessert! What a wonderful surprise will be waiting for you and your family when you pull it from the oven—maybe tonight! ☻ Serves 8

> 1½ cups Bisquick Reduced Fat Baking Mix
>
> 2 tablespoons Brown Sugar Twin
>
> ½ teaspoon ground nutmeg
>
> ⅔ cup skim milk
>
> 1 tablespoon + 1 teaspoon reduced-calorie margarine, melted
>
> 2 cups (one 16-ounce can) apricot halves, packed in fruit juice, coarsely chopped and undrained

Preheat oven to 400 degrees. Spray an 8-by-8-inch baking dish with butter-flavored cooking spray. In a large bowl, combine baking mix, Brown Sugar Twin, and nutmeg. Add skim milk and margarine. Mix well to combine. Spread mixture evenly into prepared baking dish. Pour undrained apricots evenly over top. Bake for 25 to 30 minutes. Place baking dish on a wire rack and let set for at least 4 minutes. Cut into 8 servings. Good warm or cold.

HINT: Great served warm with Wells' Blue Bunny sugar- and fat-free ice cream or any sugar- and fat-free ice cream.

Each serving equals:

HE: 1 Bread • ½ Fruit • ¼ Fat • 9 Optional Calories

130 Calories • 2 gm Fat • 3 gm Protein •
25 gm Carbohydrate • 269 mg Sodium •
51 mg Calcium • 1 gm Fiber

DIABETIC: 1 Starch • ½ Fruit • ½ Fat

Winter Banana Split Dessert

Cliff didn't want to wait until summer for a banana split dessert. I figured this layered pudding treat would satisfy my truck-drivin' man—and I was right!   ☻   Serves 8

> 1 (4-serving) package JELL-O sugar-free strawberry-banana gelatin
> 1 cup boiling water
> 2 cups cold water ☆
> 1 cup (one 8-ounce can) crushed pineapple, packed in fruit juice, undrained
> 1 cup (1 medium) diced banana
> 2 cups frozen unsweetened whole strawberries
> 1 (4-serving) package JELL-O sugar-free instant banana cream pudding mix
> ⅔ cup Carnation Nonfat Dry Milk Powder
> ½ cup Cool Whip Free
> 2 tablespoons (½ ounce) chopped pecans
> 1 tablespoon (¼ ounce) mini chocolate chips

In a medium bowl, combine dry gelatin and boiling water. Mix well to dissolve gelatin. Stir in ¾ cup cold water and undrained pineapple. Add banana and strawberries. Mix well to combine. Pour mixture into an 8-by-8-inch dish. Refrigerate until firm, about 3 hours. In a large bowl, combine dry pudding mix, dry milk powder, and remaining 1¼ cups water. Mix well using a wire whisk. Blend in Cool Whip Free. Spread pudding mixture evenly over gelatin mixture. Sprinkle pecans and chocolate chips evenly over top. Refrigerate for at least 15 minutes. Cut into 8 pieces.

Each serving equals:

HE: ¾ Fruit • ¼ Skim Milk • ¼ Fat • ¼ Slider • 10 Optional Calories

114 Calories • 2 gm Fat • 3 gm Protein •
21 gm Carbohydrate • 231 mg Sodium •
80 mg Calcium • 1 gm Fiber

DIABETIC: 1 Fruit • ½ Fat

Apple-Walnut Harvest Dessert

I love layering flavors in Healthy Exchanges recipes, so you never have to feel as if you're "settling" for something less than um-um-good! By using apple juice as my pudding liquid, then adding apples and apple pie spice, I tripled the taste—and the fun!

○ Serves 8

> 12 (2½-inch) cinnamon graham cracker squares ☆
> 1 (4-serving) package JELL-O sugar-free vanilla cook-and-serve
>   pudding mix
> 2 cups unsweetened apple juice ☆
> 2 cups (4 small) cored, unpeeled, and chopped cooking apples
> 1 teaspoon apple pie spice
> ¼ cup (1 ounce) chopped walnuts ☆
> 1 (4-serving) package JELL-O sugar-free instant vanilla pudding
>   mix
> ⅔ cup Carnation Nonfat Dry Milk Powder
> ½ cup Cool Whip Free

Layer 9 graham crackers in a 9-by-9-inch cake pan. In a large saucepan, combine dry cook-and-serve pudding mix and 1 cup apple juice. Stir in apples and apple pie spice. Cook over medium heat until mixture thickens and apples become soft, stirring often. Remove from heat. Stir in 2 tablespoons walnuts. Carefully spoon hot mixture evenly over graham crackers. Refrigerate for at least 30 minutes. In a large bowl, combine dry instant pudding mix, dry milk powder, and remaining 1 cup apple juice. Mix well using a wire whisk. Blend in Cool Whip Free. Evenly spread topping mixture over apple filling. Crush remaining 3 graham crackers. In a small bowl, combine cracker crumbs and remaining 2 tablespoons walnuts. Evenly sprinkle crumb mixture over top. Refrigerate for at least 1 hour. Cut into 8 servings.

HINT: A self-seal sandwich bag works great for crushing graham
    crackers.

Each serving equals:

HE: 1 Fruit • ½ Bread • ¼ Skim Milk • ¼ Fat • ¼ Slider • 17 Optional Calories

---

143 Calories • 3 gm Fat • 3 gm Protein • 26 gm Carbohydrate • 292 mg Sodium • 79 mg Calcium • 1 gm Fiber

---

DIABETIC: 1 Fruit • 1 Starch/Carbohydrate

Blueberry Dessert Pizza

It'd be perfect for the Fourth of July, but I think a festive "blue" dessert will be welcome just about any time at all! Imagine the applause you'll receive from a picnic table full of kids when you bring out this colorful delight.   ☉   Serves 8

1 (8-ounce) can Pillsbury Reduced Fat Crescent Rolls
1 (8-ounce) package Philadelphia fat-free cream cheese
½ cup Cool Whip Free
1 teaspoon coconut extract
1 (4-serving) package JELL-O sugar-free vanilla cook-and-serve
    pudding mix
1 (4-serving) package JELL-O sugar-free lemon gelatin
1 cup water
3 cups frozen unsweetened blueberries
2 tablespoons flaked coconut

Preheat oven to 415 degrees. Spray a rimmed 10-by-15-inch baking sheet with butter-flavored cooking spray. Gently pat crescent rolls into pan, being sure to seal perforations. Bake for 8 to 10 minutes or until lightly browned. Place baking sheet on a wire rack and let set for 10 minutes. In a medium bowl, stir cream cheese with a spoon until soft. Stir in Cool Whip Free and coconut extract. Spread cream cheese mixture evenly over cooled crust. Refrigerate while preparing topping. In a medium saucepan, combine dry pudding mix, dry gelatin, and water. Cook over medium heat until mixture thickens and starts to boil, stirring often. Remove from heat. Gently stir in frozen blueberries. Place pan on a wire rack and let set for 5 minutes. Evenly spoon blueberry mixture over cream cheese mixture. Refrigerate for at least 1 hour. Just before serving, sprinkle coconut evenly over top. Cut into 8 pieces.

HINT: Do not use inexpensive rolls, as they don't cover the pan properly.

Each serving equals:

HE: 1 Bread • ½ Protein • ½ Fruit • ¼ Slider • 6 Optional Calories

178 Calories • 6 gm Fat • 7 gm Protein • 24 gm Carbohydrate • 546 mg Sodium • 3 mg Calcium • 1 gm Fiber

DIABETIC: 1 Starch • 1 Fat • ½ Meat • ½ Fruit

Sunshine Pudding Tarts

I'm fond of saying that a day without dessert is a day when the sun doesn't shine, and these little tarts will brighten even the cloudiest day! I created this using plain graham crackers, but you could vary this dish by making it with any flavor you like.

○ Serves 6

> 1 (4-serving) package JELL-O sugar-free instant vanilla
>   pudding mix
> 1 (4-serving) package JELL-O sugar-free orange gelatin
> ⅔ cup Carnation Nonfat Dry Milk Powder
> 1½ cups water
> ¾ cup Cool Whip Free ☆
> 1 (6-single serve) package Keebler graham cracker crusts
> 2 tablespoons purchased graham cracker crumbs or
>   2 (2½-inch) graham cracker squares, made into crumbs

In a large bowl, combine dry pudding mix, dry gelatin, dry milk powder, and water. Mix well using a wire whisk. Blend in ¼ cup Cool Whip Free. Evenly spoon pudding mixture into graham cracker crusts. Refrigerate for at least 30 minutes. Just before serving, top each with 1 tablespoon Cool Whip Free and sprinkle 1 teaspoon graham cracker crumbs over top.

Each serving equals:

HE: ½ Bread • ⅓ Skim Milk • 1 Slider •
13 Optional Calories

186 Calories • 6 gm Fat • 5 gm Protein •
28 gm Carbohydrate • 467 mg Sodium •
93 mg Calcium • 1 gm Fiber

DIABETIC: 1½ Starch/Carbohydrate • 1 Fat

Steve's Coconut-Banana Cream Pie

Is there a man anywhere who isn't a fan of cream pie? I don't think I've ever met one who wasn't! This recipe doubles the flavor and the fun by doubling up on the banana and coconut ingredients. Try it on a man sometime soon!   ☻   Serves 8

1 cup (1 medium) sliced
    banana
1 (6-ounce) Keebler shortbread
    piecrust
2 (4-serving) packages JELL-O
    sugar-free instant banana
    cream pudding mix ☆

1⅓ cups Carnation Nonfat
    Dry Milk Powder ☆
2⅓ cups water ☆
½ cup Cool Whip Free
1 teaspoon coconut extract
2 tablespoons flaked coconut

Arrange banana in bottom of piecrust. In a large bowl, combine 1 package dry pudding mix, ⅔ cup dry milk powder, and 1⅓ cups water. Mix well using a wire whisk. Spread mixture evenly over banana. Refrigerate while preparing topping. In the same bowl, combine remaining dry pudding mix, remaining ⅔ cup dry milk powder, and remaining 1 cup water. Mix well using a wire whisk. Blend in Cool Whip Free and coconut extract. Spread topping mixture evenly over set filling. Evenly sprinkle coconut over top. Refrigerate for at least 1 hour. Cut into 8 pieces.

HINT: To prevent banana from turning brown, mix with 1 teaspoon lemon juice or sprinkle with Fruit Fresh.

Each serving equals:

HE: ½ Skim Milk • ½ Bread • ¼ Fruit • 1 Slider •
6 Optional Calories

197 Calories • 5 gm Fat • 5 gm Protein •
33 gm Carbohydrate • 544 mg Sodium •
140 mg Calcium • 1 gm Fiber

DIABETIC: 1½ Starch/Carbohydrate • 1 Fat •
½ Skim Milk

Car Guys Rhubarb-Pineapple Cream Pie

Here's another man-pleasing concoction that is just jam-packed with goodies! Those little marshmallows will appeal to kids from 2 to 92!   ☻   Serves 8

> 2 cups finely chopped fresh or frozen rhubarb
> ¾ cup water
> 1 cup (one 8-ounce can) crushed pineapple, packed in fruit juice, undrained
> 1 (4-serving) package JELL-O sugar-free strawberry gelatin
> 1 (4-serving) package JELL-O sugar-free vanilla cook-and-serve pudding mix
> 1 cup Cool Whip Free
> ½ cup (1 ounce) miniature marshmallows
> 1 (6-ounce) Keebler graham cracker piecrust
> 2 tablespoons purchased graham cracker crumbs or 2 (2½-inch) graham cracker squares, made into crumbs
> 2 tablespoons (½ ounce) chopped pecans

In a medium saucepan, combine rhubarb and water. Cover and cook over medium heat for 6 to 8 minutes or until rhubarb is tender. Stir in undrained pineapple. Add dry gelatin and dry pudding mix. Mix well to combine. Continue cooking for 5 minutes or until mixture thickens and begins to boil, stirring often. Place saucepan on a wire rack and allow to cool for 30 minutes, stirring occasionally. Add Cool Whip Free and marshmallows. Mix gently to combine. Spread mixture into piecrust. Evenly sprinkle cracker crumbs and pecans over top. Refrigerate for at least 2 hours. Cut into 8 pieces.

HINT: A self-seal sandwich bag works great for crushing graham crackers.

Each serving equals:

HE: ½ Bread • ½ Vegetable • ¼ Fruit • ¼ Fat •
1 Slider • 13 Optional Calories

186 Calories • 6 gm Fat • 2 gm Protein •
31 gm Carbohydrate • 181 mg Sodium •
32 mg Calcium • 1 gm Fiber

DIABETIC: 1½ Starch /Carbohydrate • 1 Fat • ½ Fruit

Strawberry Romanoff–Coconut Pie

I admit it, I created this recipe to please ME! And why not? Who knows better what I like than I do? One taste will convince you that strawberries and coconut are a marriage made in Healthy Exchanges heaven! ☺ Serves 8

4 cups sliced fresh strawberries
1 (6-ounce) Keebler graham
    cracker piecrust
1 (4-serving) package JELL-O
    sugar-free vanilla cook-
    and-serve pudding mix
1 (4-serving) package JELL-O
    sugar-free strawberry
    gelatin

1 cup unsweetened orange
    juice
½ cup + 1 teaspoon water ☆
1½ teaspoons coconut
    extract ☆
¾ cup Cool Whip Free
2 to 3 drops red food coloring
2 tablespoons flaked coconut

Layer strawberries in bottom of piecrust. In a medium saucepan, combine dry pudding mix, dry gelatin, orange juice, and ½ cup water. Cook over medium heat until mixture thickens and starts to boil, stirring often. Remove from heat and stir in 1 teaspoon coconut extract. Spoon hot mixture evenly over strawberries. Refrigerate for at least 2 hours. In a small bowl, combine Cool Whip Free and remaining ½ teaspoon coconut extract. Spread topping mixture evenly over strawberry filling. In a small bowl, combine remaining 1 teaspoon water and red food coloring. Gently stir coconut into mixture to color. Place coconut on waxed paper and allow to dry for about 5 minutes. Evenly sprinkle coconut over topping mixture. Refrigerate for at least 10 minutes. Cut into 8 pieces.

Each serving equals:

HE: ¾ Fruit • ½ Bread • 1 Slider

174 Calories • 6 gm Fat • 2 gm Protein •
28 gm Carbohydrate • 228 mg Sodium •
13 mg Calcium • 2 gm Fiber

DIABETIC: 1 Fruit • 1 Starch • 1 Fat

Maple "Ice Cream" Pumpkin Pie ❄

You don't need an ice cream freezer to stir up this chilly charmer! You'll love this unusual recipe so much, you may have to buy stock in a pumpkin farm.   ○   Serves 8

> 2 cups (one 15-ounce can) pumpkin
> ½ cup Cary's Sugar Free Maple Syrup
> 1 (4-serving) package JELL-O sugar-free instant butterscotch
>   pudding mix
> ⅔ cup Carnation Nonfat Dry Milk Powder
> 1 cup Cool Whip Free
> ½ cup (2 ounces) chopped walnuts
> 1 (6-ounce) Keebler graham cracker piecrust

In a large bowl, combine pumpkin and maple syrup. Add dry pudding mix and dry milk powder. Mix well using a wire whisk. Blend in Cool Whip Free and walnuts. Evenly spread mixture into piecrust. Cover and freeze for at least 4 hours. Remove from freezer at least 15 minutes before serving. Cut into 8 pieces.

Each serving equals:

HE: ½ Bread • ½ Fat • ½ Vegetable • ¼ Skim Milk • ¼ Protein • 1 Slider • 8 Optional Calories

225 Calories • 9 gm Fat • 4 gm Protein • 32 gm Carbohydrate • 378 mg Sodium • 92 mg Calcium • 2 gm Fiber

DIABETIC: 1½ Starch/Carbohydrate • 1 Fat • ½ Vegetable

Easy Pumpkin Raisin Pie

If you've never made a pie in the microwave, here's your chance! With the help of your not-so-silent partner, the blender, you've got a spectacularly easy dessert in no time at all. ● Serves 6

> 2 cups (one 15-ounce can) pumpkin
>
> 1½ cups (one 12-ounce can) Carnation Evaporated Skim Milk
>
> 2 eggs or equivalent in egg substitute
>
> ½ cup + 1 tablespoon Bisquick Reduced Fat Baking Mix
>
> ½ cup pourable Sugar Twin
>
> 1 teaspoon pumpkin pie spice
>
> 2 teaspoons vanilla extract
>
> ¾ cup raisins
>
> 6 tablespoons Cool Whip Lite

Spray a 9-inch glass pie plate with butter-flavored cooking spray. In a blender container, combine pumpkin, evaporated skim milk, eggs, baking mix, Sugar Twin, pumpkin pie spice, and vanilla extract. Cover and process on BLEND for 60 seconds. Pour mixture into prepared pie plate. Evenly sprinkle raisins over top. Microwave on MEDIUM (50% power) for 15 to 20 minutes, turning plate after every 5 minutes, or until edges are set but center is still slightly soft. Place pie plate on a wire rack and allow to cool for at least 30 minutes. Cut into 6 pieces. When serving, top each piece with 1 tablespoon Cool Whip Lite.

Each serving equals:

HE: 1 Fruit • ⅔ Vegetable • ½ Skim Milk •
½ Bread • ⅓ Protein (limited) • 18 Optional Calories

215 Calories • 3 gm Fat • 9 gm Protein •
38 gm Carbohydrate • 234 mg Sodium •
233 mg Calcium • 3 gm Fiber

DIABETIC: 1 Fruit • 1 Starch/Carbohydrate •
½ Skim Milk

Butterscotch Raisin
Sour Cream Pie

Raisin pies are a Midwest staple at bake sales and potlucks, so I'm always thinking up new ways to feed that happy hunger! This one is especially creamy and rich, so enjoy!   ○   Serves 8

> 1 (4-serving) package JELL-O sugar-free instant butterscotch
>   pudding mix
> ⅔ cup Carnation Nonfat Dry Milk Powder
> 1½ cups water
> ½ cup Land O Lakes no-fat sour cream
> ¼ teaspoon ground cinnamon
> 1 cup raisins ☆
> 1 (6-ounce) Keebler graham cracker piecrust
> ½ cup Cool Whip Lite

In a large bowl, combine dry pudding mix, dry milk powder, and water. Mix well using a wire whisk. Fold in sour cream and cinnamon. Reserve 8 raisins. Fold remaining raisins into pudding mixture. Spread mixture evenly into piecrust. Refrigerate for 10 minutes. Drop Cool Whip Lite by tablespoonful over set filling to form 8 dollops. Garnish each dollop with 1 raisin. Refrigerate for at least 1 hour. Cut into 8 pieces.

HINT: To plump up raisins without "cooking," place in a glass
    measuring cup and microwave on HIGH for 20 seconds.

Each serving equals:

HE: 1 Fruit • ½ Bread • ¼ Skim Milk • 1 Slider •
7 Optional Calories

214 Calories • 6 gm Fat • 4 gm Protein •
36 gm Carbohydrate • 358 mg Sodium •
95 mg Calcium • 1 gm Fiber

DIABETIC: 1½ Starch/Carbohydrate • 1 Fruit • 1 Fat

Regal Cherry Meringue Pie

My son James is a terrific entrepreneur who's created so many great products to make caring for your children easier. I may be prejudiced (I *am* his mother), but I think he's a king among men. James, this one's for you!   ☻   Serves 8

> 2 cups (one 16-ounce can) tart red cherries, packed in water, undrained
> 1 (4-serving) package JELL-O sugar-free vanilla cook-and-serve pudding mix
> 1 (4-serving) package JELL-O sugar-free cherry gelatin
> ½ cup water
> 1½ teaspoons almond extract ☆
> 6 egg whites
> ½ cup pourable Sugar Twin
> 2 tablespoons (½ ounce) chopped almonds
> 1 (6-ounce) Keebler shortbread piecrust

Preheat oven to 350 degrees. In a medium saucepan, combine undrained cherries, dry pudding mix, dry gelatin, and water. Mix well to combine. Cook over medium heat until mixture thickens and starts to boil, stirring constantly and being careful not to crush cherries. Remove from heat. Stir in 1 teaspoon almond extract. Place saucepan on a wire rack and allow to cool for 5 minutes. Meanwhile, in a large bowl, beat egg whites with an electric mixer on HIGH until soft peaks form. Add remaining ½ teaspoon almond extract and Sugar Twin. Continue beating until stiff peaks form. Stir in almonds. Spoon partially cooled cherry mixture into piecrust. Spread meringue mixture evenly over filling, being sure to seal completely to edges of piecrust. Bake for 12 to 15 minutes or until meringue starts to turn golden brown. Place pie plate on a wire rack and allow to cool 15 minutes. Refrigerate for at least 1 hour. Cut into 8 pieces.

HINTS: 1. Egg whites beat best at room temperature.
2. Meringue pie cuts easily if you dip a sharp knife in warm water before slicing.

Each serving equals:

HE: ½ Bread • ½ Fruit • ¼ Protein • 1 Slider

161 Calories • 5 gm Fat • 5 gm Protein •
24 gm Carbohydrate • 225 mg Sodium •
14 mg Calcium • 1 gm Fiber

DIABETIC: 1 Starch /Carbohydrate • 1 Fat • ½ Fruit

Angie's Creamy Cheesecake

When Tommy brought Angie home for the first time, I knew I would soon be losing my youngest child to another woman! My son chose a wonderful girl for his bride, and it's been such a joy to have her in our family.   ☻   Serves 8

> 2 (8-ounce) packages Philadelphia fat-free cream cheese
> 1 (4-serving) package JELL-O sugar-free instant vanilla
>   pudding mix
> ⅔ cup Carnation Nonfat Dry Milk Powder
> 1½ cups water ☆
> 1 teaspoon vanilla extract
> ½ cup Cool Whip Free
> 1 (6-ounce) Keebler graham cracker piecrust
> 1 (4-serving) package JELL-O sugar-free vanilla cook-and-serve
>   pudding mix
> 1 (4-serving) package JELL-O sugar-free cherry gelatin
> 2 cups (one 16-ounce can) tart red cherries, packed in water,
>   drained and ½ cup liquid reserved ☆

In a large bowl, stir cream cheese with a spoon until soft. Add dry instant pudding mix, dry milk powder, and 1 cup water. Mix well using a wire whisk. Blend in vanilla extract and Cool Whip Free. Evenly spread mixture into piecrust. Refrigerate for 2 hours. Meanwhile, in a medium saucepan, combine dry cook-and-serve pudding mix, dry gelatin, reserved cherry liquid, and remaining ½ cup water. Cook over medium heat until mixture thickens and starts to boil, stirring constantly. Remove from heat. Gently stir in cherries. Place saucepan on a wire rack and allow mixture to cool for 15 minutes, stirring occasionally. Transfer mixture to a bowl, cover, and refrigerate until ready to serve. When serving, cut cheesecake into 8 pieces and spoon about ¼ cup cherry mixture over each piece.

Each serving equals:

HE: 1 Protein • ½ Bread • ½ Fruit • ¼ Skim Milk •
1 Slider • 5 Optional Calories

---

230 Calories • 6 gm Fat • 12 gm Protein •
32 gm Carbohydrate • 764 mg Sodium •
76 mg Calcium • 1 gm Fiber

DIABETIC: 1½ Starch/Carbohydrate • 1 Meat • 1 Fat •
½ Fruit

White Chocolate Raspberry Cheesecake

Sometimes just the name of a recipe will get my mouth watering, and this is one of those! White chocolate has always had a reputation for being a luxury food, something served only for very special occasions. But thanks to the folks at JELL-O, we can enjoy this dazzling flavor treat as often as we like! ☺ Serves 8

> 2 (8-ounce) packages Philadelphia fat-free cream cheese
> 1 (4-serving) package JELL-O sugar-free instant white chocolate pudding mix
> ⅔ cup Carnation Nonfat Dry Milk Powder
> 2 cups water ☆
> ¼ cup Cool Whip Free
> 1 (6-ounce) Keebler chocolate piecrust
> 1 (4-serving) package JELL-O sugar-free raspberry gelatin
> 1 (4-serving) package JELL-O sugar-free vanilla cook-and-serve pudding mix
> 1½ cups frozen unsweetened raspberries
> 2 tablespoons (½ ounce) mini chocolate chips

In a large bowl, stir cream cheese with a spoon until soft. Add dry instant pudding mix, dry milk powder, and 1 cup water. Mix well using a wire whisk. Blend in Cool Whip Free. Spread mixture evenly into piecrust. Refrigerate. Meanwhile, in a medium saucepan, combine dry gelatin, dry cook-and-serve pudding mix, and remaining 1 cup water. Cook over medium heat until mixture thickens and starts to boil, stirring often. Remove from heat. Gently stir in raspberries. Place saucepan on a wire rack and let set for 10 minutes, stirring occasionally. Evenly spoon raspberry mixture over cream cheese mixture. Refrigerate for at least 1 hour. Just before serving, evenly sprinkle chocolate chips over top. Cut into 8 pieces.

Each serving equals:

HE: 1 Protein • ½ Bread • ¼ Skim Milk • ¼ Fruit •
1 Slider • 16 Optional Calories

213 Calories • 5 gm Fat • 12 gm Protein •
30 gm Carbohydrate • 664 mg Sodium •
75 mg Calcium • 1 gm Fiber

DIABETIC: 1½ Starch/Carbohydrate • 1 Meat • 1 Fat

Black Tie Chocolate Cheesecake

When it's time to party, why not pull out all the stops and really "dress" for the occasion? Here's an elegant, rich dessert that is as far from the concept of diet food as any cheesecake could be.

☻ Serves 8

¾ cup all-purpose flour

2 tablespoons unsweetened cocoa

½ cup pourable Sugar Twin

½ teaspoon baking powder

½ teaspoon baking soda

¼ cup Dannon plain fat-free yogurt

3 tablespoons Kraft fat-free mayonnaise

2½ cups water ☆

1 teaspoon vanilla extract

1 (8-ounce) package Philadelphia fat-free cream cheese

1 (4-serving) package JELL-O sugar-free instant chocolate fudge pudding mix

1⅓ cups Carnation Nonfat Dry Milk Powder☆

¾ cup Cool Whip Free ☆

1 (4-serving) package JELL-O sugar-free instant white chocolate pudding mix

2 tablespoons (½ ounce) mini chocolate chips

Preheat oven to 350 degrees. Spray a 10-inch deep dish pie plate with butter-flavored cooking spray. In a large bowl, combine flour, cocoa, Sugar Twin, baking powder, and baking soda. In a small bowl, combine yogurt, mayonnaise, ½ cup water, and vanilla extract. Add yogurt mixture to flour mixture. Mix gently just to combine. Spread batter into prepared pie plate. Bake for 8 to 10 minutes or until a toothpick inserted in center comes out clean. (Surface will not be smooth.) Place pie plate on a wire rack and allow to cool for 15 minutes. After crust has cooled, in a large bowl, stir cream cheese with a spoon until soft. Add dry chocolate fudge pudding mix, ⅔ cup dry milk powder, and 1 cup water. Mix well using a wire whisk. Blend in ¼ cup Cool Whip Free. Spread mixture evenly over cooled crust. Refrigerate while preparing topping. In a medium bowl, combine dry white chocolate pudding mix, remaining ⅔ cup dry milk powder, and remaining 1 cup water. Mix well using a wire whisk. Blend in remaining ½ cup Cool Whip Free. Spread topping mixture evenly over chocolate layer. Evenly sprinkle chocolate chips over top. Refrigerate for at least 1 hour. Cut into 8 pieces.

Each serving equals:

HE: ½ Skim Milk • ½ Bread • ½ Protein • ¾ Slider • 12 Optional Calories

---

157 Calories • 1 gm Fat • 10 gm Protein • 27 gm Carbohydrate • 583 mg Sodium • 160 mg Calcium • 1 gm Fiber

---

DIABETIC: 1½ Starch/Carbohydrate • ½ Skim Milk • ½ Meat

Holiday Orange Cheesecake
with Cranberry Glaze

My friend Barbara told me about a sorbet flavor she'd enjoyed that combined the tartness of cranberry with the lush sweetness of orange. This is for you, B!   ☻   Serves 8

> 1 (4-serving) package JELL-O sugar-free vanilla
>   cook-and-serve pudding mix
> 1 cup Ocean Spray reduced-calorie cranberry juice
>   cocktail
> 1 cup fresh or frozen cranberries
> 2 (8-ounce) packages Philadelphia fat-free
>   cream cheese
> 1 (4-serving) package JELL-O sugar-free instant
>   vanilla pudding mix
> ⅔ cup Carnation Nonfat Dry Milk Powder
> 1 cup unsweetened orange juice
> ¼ cup Cool Whip Free
> 1 (6-ounce) Keebler graham cracker piecrust
> 2 tablespoons (½ ounce) chopped pecans

In a medium saucepan, combine dry cook-and-serve pudding mix, cranberry juice cocktail, and cranberries. Cook over medium heat until mixture thickens and cranberries soften, stirring often. Place saucepan on a wire rack and allow to cool for 15 minutes, stirring occasionally. Meanwhile, in a large bowl, stir cream cheese with a spoon until soft. Add dry instant pudding mix, dry milk powder, and orange juice. Mix well using a wire whisk. Blend in Cool Whip Free. Spread mixture evenly into piecrust. Evenly spread cooled cranberry mixture over cream cheese filling. Sprinkle pecans evenly over top. Refrigerate for at least 2 hours. Cut into 8 pieces.

Each serving equals:

HE: 1 Protein • ½ Bread • ½ Fruit • ¼ Skim Milk • ¼ Fat • ¾ Slider • 16 Optional Calories

226 Calories • 6 gm Fat • 11 gm Protein • 32 gm Carbohydrate • 734 mg Sodium • 73 mg Calcium • 1 gm Fiber

DIABETIC: 1½ Starch/Carbohydrate • 1 Meat • ½ Fruit • ½ Fat

Heart's Desire Apple Pie

If your idea of happiness is pie a la mode, you might find your heart's desire in this delectable recipe! How can I bake a pie with ice cream in it, without making a mess of my oven? Try it and see!

◑ Serves 8

4 cups (8 small) peeled and sliced cooking apples
1 (6-ounce) Keebler graham cracker piecrust
1 cup Wells' Blue Bunny sugar- and fat-free vanilla ice cream or
    any sugar- and fat-free ice cream, softened
½ cup pourable Sugar Twin
6 tablespoons all-purpose flour
1 teaspoon apple pie spice
6 tablespoons purchased graham cracker crumbs or 6 (2½-inch)
    graham cracker squares, made into crumbs

Preheat oven to 425 degrees. Evenly arrange apples in bottom of piecrust. In a medium bowl, combine ice cream, Sugar Twin, flour, and apple pie spice. Spoon mixture evenly over apples. Evenly sprinkle graham cracker crumbs over top. Bake for 15 minutes. Reduce heat to 350 degrees. Continue baking for 45 minutes. Place pie plate on a wire rack and allow to cool completely. Cut into 8 pieces.

Each serving equals:

HE: 1 Bread • 1 Fruit • ¾ Slider •
19 Optional Calories

205 Calories • 5 gm Fat • 3 gm Protein •
37 gm Carbohydrate • 142 mg Sodium •
35 mg Calcium • 2 gm Fiber

DIABETIC: 1 Starch • 1 Fruit • 1 Fat

Lemon Cakes with Blueberry Cream Sauce

I've always been a fan of blueberry and lemon served together, maybe because lemon brings out the best in fresh berries! This dessert is both pretty to look at and scrumptious to savor. It's perfect for a summer supper or even for a late brunch. ◐ Serves 4

> ½ cup Cool Whip Free
> 2 tablespoons blueberry spreadable fruit
> 1½ cups fresh blueberries
> ¾ cup Bisquick Reduced Fat Baking Mix
> ⅓ cup Carnation Nonfat Dry Milk Powder
> 1 (4-serving) package JELL-O sugar-free lemon gelatin
> 2 tablespoons Land O Lakes no-fat sour cream
> ⅓ cup Diet Mountain Dew

Preheat oven to 400 degrees. Spray 4 wells of a muffin pan with butter-flavored cooking spray. In a medium bowl, combine Cool Whip Free and spreadable fruit. Gently stir in blueberries. Cover and refrigerate. Meanwhile, in a large bowl, combine baking mix, dry milk powder, and dry gelatin. Add sour cream and Diet Mountain Dew. Mix well to combine. Evenly spoon mixture into prepared muffin wells. Bake for 8 to 12 minutes or until golden brown. Place muffin pan on a wire rack and let set for at least 10 minutes. For each serving, place 1 cake on a dessert plate and spoon about ½ cup blueberry cream sauce over top.

HINT: Fill unused muffin wells with water. It protects the muffin pan and ensures even baking.

Each serving equals:

HE: 1 Bread • 1 Fruit • ¼ Skim Milk • ¼ Slider • 5 Optional Calories

178 Calories • 2 gm Fat • 5 gm Protein • 35 gm Carbohydrate • 402 mg Sodium • 99 mg Calcium • 2 gm Fiber

DIABETIC: 1½ Starch/Carbohydrate • 1 Fat

Fresh Applesauce Spice Cake

This sweetly spicy apple "triple threat" is one of those cakes that tastes great the day you bake it, but even better the next day, and the next. It freezes beautifully, so you may want to keep one on hand for unexpected company. ☻ Serves 8

1½ cups all-purpose flour
½ cup pourable Sugar Twin
2 tablespoons Brown Sugar
   Twin
1 teaspoon baking soda
1 teaspoon baking powder
1 teaspoon apple pie spice
½ cup unsweetened applesauce

½ cup unsweetened apple juice
1 egg or equivalent in egg
   substitute
2 cups (4 small) cored, peeled
   and finely chopped
   cooking apples
¼ cup (1 ounce) chopped
   walnuts

Preheat oven to 350 degrees. Spray a 9-by-9-inch cake pan with butter-flavored cooking spray. In a large bowl, combine flour, Sugar Twin, Brown Sugar Twin, baking soda, baking powder, and apple pie spice. In a small bowl, combine applesauce, apple juice, and egg. Add applesauce mixture to flour mixture. Mix gently just to combine. Fold in apples and walnuts. Spread batter into prepared cake pan. Bake for 30 to 35 minutes or until a toothpick inserted in center comes out clean. Place cake pan on a wire rack and let set for at least 15 minutes. Cut into 8 pieces.

Each serving equals:

HE: 1 Bread • ¾ Fruit • ¼ Fat • ¼ Protein •
7 Optional Calories

147 Calories • 3 gm Fat • 4 gm Protein •
26 gm Carbohydrate • 233 mg Sodium •
13 mg Calcium • 2 gm Fiber

DIABETIC: 1 Starch • 1 Fruit

Dixie Chocolate Mayonnaise Cake

I remember when I first heard the term "mayonnaise cake" and thought, that sounds so strange! Then I remember that mayonnaise is really just eggs and oil, which makes it a perfect shortening agent for baking. What a tasty, moist delight this cake is!   ☽   Serves 8

    1½ cups all-purpose flour
    ¾ cup pourable Sugar Twin
    ¼ cup unsweetened cocoa
    1½ teaspoons baking soda
    ¾ cup Kraft fat-free mayonnaise
    ¾ cup + 2 tablespoons water
    2 teaspoons vanilla extract
    2 tablespoons (½ ounce) chopped pecans
    ½ cup apricot spreadable fruit

Preheat oven to 350 degrees. Spray a 9-by-9-inch cake pan with butter-flavored cooking spray. In a large bowl, combine flour, Sugar Twin, cocoa, and baking soda. Add mayonnaise, water, and vanilla extract. Mix gently just to combine. Stir in pecans. Spread batter into prepared cake pan. Bake for 25 to 30 minutes or until a toothpick inserted in center comes out clean. Place cake pan on a wire rack. In a small bowl, stir spreadable fruit with a spoon to soften and evenly spread over warm cake. Continue cooling for at least 15 minutes. Cut into 8 pieces.

Each serving equals:

HE: 1 Bread • 1 Fruit • ¼ Fat • ¼ Slider • 11 Optional Calories

162 Calories • 2 gm Fat • 3 gm Protein • 33 gm Carbohydrate • 432 mg Sodium • 7 mg Calcium • 2 gm Fiber

DIABETIC: 1½ Starch/Carbohydrate • 1 Fruit

Luck of the Irish Dream Cake

Remember those buttons and T-shirts you often see on St. Patrick's Day? "When you're in love, the whole world is Irish!" Well, even if you never make it overseas to kiss the Blarney Stone for luck, here's a dessert that will convince you with just one taste that you're lucky too!   ◐   Serves 12

> 1⅓ cups Carnation Nonfat Dry Milk Powder ☆
> 2 cups water ☆
> 2 teaspoons white vinegar
> 1½ cups all-purpose flour
> ½ cup pourable Sugar Twin
> 1 teaspoon baking powder
> 1 teaspoon baking soda
> ½ cup Kraft fat-free mayonnaise
> ⅓ cup Dannon plain fat-free yogurt
> 2 teaspoons vanilla extract
> 6 to 8 drops green food coloring
> 1 (4-serving) package JELL-O sugar-free instant pistachio
>   pudding mix
> 1 cup Cool Whip Free

Preheat oven to 350 degrees. Spray a 9-by-13-inch cake pan with butter-flavored cooking spray. In a small bowl, combine ⅔ cup dry milk powder, 1 cup water, and vinegar. Set aside. In a large bowl, combine flour, Sugar Twin, baking powder, and baking soda. To milk mixture, add mayonnaise, yogurt, vanilla extract, and green food coloring. Mix well to combine. Add milk mixture to flour mixture. Mix gently just to combine. Spread batter into prepared cake pan. Bake for 18 to 22 minutes or until a toothpick inserted in center comes out clean. Place cake pan on a wire rack and allow to cool completely. In a medium bowl, combine dry pudding mix, remaining ⅔ cup dry milk powder, and remaining 1 cup water. Mix well using a wire whisk. Blend in Cool Whip Free. Spread pudding mixture evenly over cooled cake. Cut into 12 pieces.

Each serving equals:

HE: ⅔ Bread • ⅓ Skim Milk • ¼ Slider •
12 Optional Calories

112 Calories • 0 gm Fat • 4 gm Protein •
24 gm Carbohydrate • 490 mg Sodium •
118 mg Calcium • 0 gm Fiber

DIABETIC: 1 Starch/Carbohydrate • ½ Skim Milk

Chocolate-Berry Roll

If you've never made a homemade "jelly roll" type cake, read the instructions carefully, but definitely give this luscious treat a try! Everyone at the table will be dazzled by the beauty and the taste.

🌑 Serves 8

> 4 eggs or equivalent in egg substitute
> 1 teaspoon vanilla extract
> ½ cup pourable Sugar Twin
> ¾ cup Aunt Jemima Reduced Calorie Pancake Mix
> 3 tablespoons unsweetened cocoa
> 2 cups whole fresh strawberries ☆
> 1 (4-serving) package JELL-O sugar-free instant white chocolate
>   pudding mix
> ⅔ cup Carnation Nonfat Dry Milk Powder
> 1 cup water
> ½ cup Cool Whip Free
> ½ cup Hershey's Lite Chocolate Syrup

Preheat oven to 400 degrees. Line a 10-by-15-inch rimmed baking sheet with wax paper and spray paper with butter-flavored cooking spray. In a large bowl, combine eggs, vanilla extract, and Sugar Twin. Mix well using an electric mixer on HIGH until mixture is fluffy. Add dry pancake mix and cocoa. Continue mixing on HIGH until well blended. Pour batter into prepared baking sheet. Bake for 6 to 8 minutes or until a toothpick inserted in center comes out clean. Place a clean cloth over top, turn baking sheet over, and gently remove cake. Carefully peel wax paper off cake. Starting at narrow end, roll cake with a clean towel inside. Allow to cool for 30 minutes. Reserve 8 whole strawberries. Finely chop remaining strawberries. In a large bowl, combine dry pudding mix, dry milk powder, and water. Mix well using a wire whisk. Blend in Cool Whip Free. Add chopped strawberries. Mix gently to combine. Carefully unroll cooled cake and remove towel. Spread pudding mixture evenly over top. Reroll. Place cake on a serving plate, seam side down, and refrigerate for at least 30 minutes. Cut into 8 pieces. When serving, top each piece with a whole strawberry and drizzle 1 tablespoon chocolate syrup over top.

Each serving equals:

HE: ½ Bread • ½ Protein (limited) • ¼ Skim Milk • ¼ Fruit • ½ Slider • 12 Optional Calories

155 Calories • 3 gm Fat • 8 gm Protein • 24 gm Carbohydrate • 375 mg Sodium • 157 mg Calcium • 3 gm Fiber

DIABETIC: 1½ Starch/Carbohydrate • ½ Meat

Carrot Cake Cookies

If you're a lover of rich, sweet carrot cake, then here's another dream-come-true to please your sweet tooth! You'll notice, of course, that I don't shout "low-fat and low-calorie," then expect you to eat *one* cookie for a serving. Instead, you get a "real world" serving of four!   ☻   Serves 8 (4 each)

1½ cups all-purpose flour
½ cup pourable Sugar Twin
2 teaspoons pumpkin pie
   spice
1 teaspoon baking powder
1 teaspoon baking soda
6 tablespoons raisins
1 cup finely grated carrots

¼ cup (1 ounce) chopped
   walnuts
½ cup unsweetened applesauce
1 egg or equivalent in egg
   substitute
2 tablespoons Kraft fat-free
   mayonnaise
½ cup water

Preheat oven to 350 degrees. Spray 3 baking sheets with butter-flavored cooking spray. In a large bowl, combine flour, Sugar Twin, pumpkin pie spice, baking powder, and baking soda. Stir in raisins, carrots, and walnuts. In a medium bowl, combine applesauce, egg, mayonnaise, and water. Add applesauce mixture to flour mixture. Mix gently just to combine. Drop batter by tablespoonful to form 32 cookies on prepared baking sheets. Flatten each cookie with a fork. Bake for 12 to 16 minutes or until cookies are lightly browned. Place baking sheets on a wire rack and let set for 5 minutes. Remove cookies from baking sheets and continue cooling on wire racks.

Each serving equals:

HE: 1 Bread • ½ Fruit • ¼ Protein • ¼ Fat •
¼ Vegetable • 9 Optional Calories

---

155 Calories • 3 gm Fat • 4 gm Protein •
28 gm Carbohydrate • 266 mg Sodium •
54 mg Calcium • 2 gm Fiber

DIABETIC: 1 Starch/Carbohydrate • ½ Fruit • ½ Fat

Raspberry Chocolate Layer Cake

Layer cake? In a healthy eating cookbook? Is that *possible?* Not only is it possible, it's downright delectable! Eating well is an important part of living well and feeling good, so I'm thrilled to offer you this magical, flavorful cake. ☻ Serves 12

> 1½ cups all-purpose flour
> ½ cup pourable Sugar Twin
> ¼ cup unsweetened cocoa
> 1 teaspoon baking soda
> 1 teaspoon baking powder
> ½ cup Dannon plain fat-free
>   yogurt
> ⅓ cup Kraft fat-free
>   mayonnaise
>
> 1 teaspoon almond extract
> ⅔ cup water
> ¾ cup raspberry spreadable
>   fruit ☆
> 2 tablespoons (½ ounce)
>   chopped almonds
> 2 tablespoons (½ ounce) mini
>   chocolate chips

Preheat oven to 350 degrees. Spray a 9-by-13-inch cake pan with butter-flavored cooking spray. In a large bowl, combine flour, Sugar Twin, cocoa, baking soda, and baking powder. In a medium bowl, combine yogurt, mayonnaise, almond extract, water, and ½ cup spreadable fruit. Add yogurt mixture to flour mixture. Mix gently just to combine. Spread batter into prepared cake pan. Bake for 20 minutes. In a small bowl, stir remaining ¼ cup spreadable fruit with a spoon until soft. Drizzle softened spread evenly over partially baked cake. Evenly sprinkle almonds and chocolate chips over top. Continue baking for 10 to 15 minutes or until a toothpick inserted in center comes out clean. Place cake pan on a wire rack and allow to cool completely. Cut into 12 pieces.

Each serving equals:

HE: 1 Fruit • ⅔ Bread • ¼ Slider •
9 Optional Calories

125 Calories • 1 gm Fat • 3 gm Protein •
26 gm Carbohydrate • 211 mg Sodium •
50 mg Calcium • 1 gm Fiber

DIABETIC: 1 Fruit • 1 Starch

This and That

Garden Vegetable Spread

Here's a savory veggie dip that is wonderful for crudités and also good for topping a baked potato! ☺ Serves 6 (¼ cup)

1 (8-ounce) package Philadelphia fat-free cream cheese
½ cup finely chopped cucumber
½ cup shredded carrots
2 tablespoons chopped green onion
1 teaspoon lemon juice
¼ teaspoon dried dill weed

In a medium bowl, stir cream cheese with a spoon until soft. Add cucumber, carrots, green onion, lemon juice, and dill weed. Mix well to combine. Cover and refrigerate for at least 1 hour. Gently stir again just before serving.

Each serving equals:

HE: ⅔ Protein • ⅓ Vegetable

36 Calories • 0 gm Fat • 6 gm Protein •
3 gm Carbohydrate • 230 mg Sodium •
5 mg Calcium • 0 gm Fiber

DIABETIC: 1 Meat

Southern Fruit Spread

Yes, you *could* spread a little diet margarine on your toast, but that wouldn't be the best you could do for yourself. Instead, enjoy something truly special in the morning, and see if you don't think this is "as good as it gets!" ☻ Serves 8 (3 tablespoons)

1 (8-ounce) package Philadelphia fat-free cream cheese
½ cup apricot spreadable fruit
¼ cup (1 ounce) chopped pecans

In a medium bowl, stir cream cheese with a spoon until soft. Add spreadable fruit and pecans. Mix gently to combine. Cover and refrigerate for at least 30 minutes. Gently stir again just before serving.

Each serving equals:

HE: 1 Fruit • ½ Protein • ½ Fat

91 Calories • 3 gm Fat • 4 gm Protein • 12 gm Carbohydrate • 170 mg Sodium • 1 mg Calcium • 0 gm Fiber

DIABETIC: 1 Fruit • ½ Meat • ½ Fat

Zucchini Marinara Sauce

This is another great solution for an abundant zucchini harvest—or just if you love that great green vegetable! Once you've tasted homemade "from scratch" sauce, you might not settle for canned spaghetti sauce again!   ☻   Serves 4 (½ cup)

2 tablespoons Kraft Fat Free Italian Dressing
4 cups sliced unpeeled zucchini
1 cup (one 8-ounce can) Hunt's Tomato Sauce
1 teaspoon pourable Sugar Twin

Pour Italian dressing into a large skillet. Stir in zucchini. Cook over medium heat for 6 to 8 minutes or until zucchini becomes soft, stirring occasionally. Add tomato sauce and Sugar Twin. Mix well to combine. Lower heat and simmer for 10 minutes, or until mixture is heated through, stirring occasionally.

Each serving equals:

HE: 3 Vegetable • 5 Optional Calories

40 Calories • 0 gm Fat • 2 gm Protein •
8 gm Carbohydrate • 481 mg Sodium •
20 mg Calcium • 3 gm Fiber

DIABETIC: 2 Vegetable

Triple Berry Freezer Jam

Last summer I kept bringing home pints of fresh berries from the farmers' market, and when I realized just how many berries I'd bought, I figured I'd better think of a way to make that pleasure last a l-o-n-g time! Even if you've never made jam, you'll feel like a kitchen whiz when you save your summer in a jar of berries!

> *3 cups sliced fresh strawberries*
> *2 cups fresh red raspberries*
> *1 cup fresh blueberries*
> *1 (4-serving) package JELL-O sugar-free lemon gelatin*
> *¼ cup pourable Sugar Twin*
> *1 pouch liquid Certo*

In a large saucepan, mash fruit with a potato masher. Stir in dry gelatin. Cook over medium heat for 5 minutes or until mixture starts to boil, stirring often. Add Sugar Twin and liquid Certo. Mix well to combine. Continue boiling for about 1 minute, stirring constantly. Pour hot mixture into containers. Let cool for at least 30 minutes. Cover and refrigerate overnight before using. Will keep up to 3 weeks in refrigerator or 6 months in the freezer.

1 tablespoon serving equals:

HE: 8 Optional Calories

8 Calories • 0 gm Fat • 0 gm Protein •
2 gm Carbohydrate • 7 mg Sodium •
4 mg Calcium • 1 gm Fiber

DIABETIC: 1 Free Food

Baby Quiche Appetizers

I believe in celebrating as many joyous occasions as you can, and I like coming up with party food that lets you eat healthy and still feel festive. These little pie-lets are a terrific choice with guests of all ages! 🔄 Serves 12 (3 each)

¾ cup (3 ounces) shredded Kraft reduced-fat Cheddar cheese

½ cup finely chopped onion

½ cup finely shredded carrots

½ cup finely chopped broccoli

1 cup skim milk

2 eggs, beaten, or equivalent in egg substitute

1 cup + 2 tablespoons Bisquick Reduced Fat Baking Mix

½ teaspoon lemon pepper

Preheat oven to 350 degrees. Spray 3 (12-hole) mini muffin pans with butter-flavored cooking spray. In a large bowl, combine Cheddar cheese, onion, carrots, and broccoli. In a blender container, combine skim milk, eggs, baking mix, and lemon pepper. Cover and process on BLEND for 30 seconds or until smooth. Add milk mixture to vegetable mixture. Mix well to combine. Evenly spoon mixture into prepared muffin pans. Bake for 18 to 22 minutes or until lightly browned. Place muffin pans on a wire rack and let set for 5 minutes. Good warm or cold.

Each serving equals:

HE: ½ Bread • ½ Protein • ¼ Vegetable • 7 Optional Calories

---

83 Calories • 3 gm Fat • 4 gm Protein • 10 gm Carbohydrate • 214 mg Sodium • 89 mg Calcium • 1 gm Fiber

---

DIABETIC: ½ Starch • ½ Meat

Apple Scrapple

For all you city dwellers, perhaps a word of explanation is in order here. "Scrapple" is farm food, a kind of cornmeal mush that's made with boiled meat scraps and served in slices, fried. Here's a much healthier version that's perfect for breakfast or brunch, with great fruit flavors and the tang of maple! *Note: You'll want to prepare this the night before since it should set for 8 hours.*   ☉   Serves 8

3 cups water
⅛ teaspoon salt
1 cup (3 ounces) dry
     Cream of Wheat
1 cup (2 small) cored,
     unpeeled, and chopped
     cooking apples

½ cup raisins
1 cup (one 8-ounce can)
     crushed pineapple, packed
     in fruit juice, drained
¼ cup pourable Sugar Twin
1 cup Cary's Sugar Free Maple
     Syrup

Spray a 9-by-5-inch loaf pan with butter-flavored cooking spray. In a medium saucepan, bring water and salt to a boil. Stir in Cream of Wheat. Cook over medium heat for 15 minutes, stirring occasionally. Add apples, raisins, pineapple, and Sugar Twin. Mix well to combine. Remove from heat and spoon mixture into prepared loaf pan. Cover and refrigerate for at least 8 hours. Cut chilled loaf into 8 even slices. Spray a griddle or skillet with butter-flavored cooking spray and brown slices about 5 minutes on each side. When serving, drizzle 2 tablespoons maple syrup over each piece.

HINT: To plump up raisins without "cooking," place in a glass measuring cup and microwave on HIGH for 20 seconds.

Each serving equals:

HE: 1 Fruit • ½ Bread • ¼ Slider • 3 Optional Calories

88 Calories • 0 gm Fat • 1 gm Protein •
21 gm Carbohydrate • 120 mg Sodium •
11 mg Calcium • 1 gm Fiber

DIABETIC: 1 Fruit • 1 Starch/Carbohydrate

Blueberry-Peach
Cobbler Muffins

Muffins are such a great mainstay for anyone committed to living healthy. They're easy to prepare, take only a little while to bake, and freeze wonderfully well. If you spend one morning on a weekend making muffins, you'll be set for days to come!

○ Serves 8

1½ cups all-purpose flour
1 (4-serving) package JELL-O sugar-free instant vanilla
*   pudding mix*
1 teaspoon baking powder
½ teaspoon baking soda
¾ cup fresh blueberries
½ cup (1 medium) peeled and diced fresh peach
¼ cup (1 ounce) chopped walnuts
¾ cup Dannon plain fat-free yogurt
2 tablespoons Kraft fat-free mayonnaise
⅓ cup Carnation Nonfat Dry Milk Powder
½ cup water
1 teaspoon coconut extract
2 tablespoons pourable Sugar Twin
1 tablespoon + 1 teaspoon flaked coconut

Preheat oven to 375 degrees. Spray 8 wells of a 12-hole muffin pan with butter-flavored cooking spray or line with paper liners. In a large bowl, combine flour, dry pudding mix, baking powder, and baking soda. Stir in blueberries, peaches, and walnuts. In a medium bowl, combine yogurt, mayonnaise, and dry milk powder. Stir in water and coconut extract. Add yogurt mixture to flour mixture. Mix gently just to combine. Evenly spoon batter into prepared muffin wells. In a small bowl, combine Sugar Twin and coconut. Sprinkle a full teaspoon over top of each muffin. Bake for 25 to 30 minutes or until a toothpick inserted in center comes out clean. Place muffin pan on a wire rack and let set for 5 minutes. Remove muffins and continue cooling on wire rack.

HINT: Fill unused muffin wells with water. It protects the muffin pan and ensures even baking.

Each serving equals:

HE: 1 Bread • ¼ Skim Milk • ¼ Fruit • ¼ Fat • ¼ Slider • 7 Optional Calories

159 Calories • 3 gm Fat • 5 gm Protein • 28 gm Carbohydrate • 416 mg Sodium • 119 mg Calcium • 2 gm Fiber

DIABETIC: 1½ Starch/Carbohydrate • ½ Fat

Baked Strawberry Toast

This creamy, fruity, "French-toast-in-the-oven" recipe will be loved by both children and adults! I could eat this for breakfast three times a week all summer long—but then, I'm a serious strawberry fan! ☻ Serves 4

8 slices reduced-calorie white bread ☆

1 (8-ounce) package Philadelphia fat-free cream cheese

½ cup pourable Sugar Twin ☆

4 cups sliced fresh strawberries ☆

⅔ cup Carnation Nonfat Dry Milk Powder

1¼ cups water ☆

2 eggs or equivalent in egg substitute

1 teaspoon almond extract

2 tablespoons (½ ounce) slivered almonds

Preheat oven to 375 degrees. Spray a 9-by-9-inch cake pan with butter-flavored cooking spray. Arrange 4 slices of bread in prepared cake pan. In a medium bowl, stir cream cheese with a spoon until soft. Stir in 2 tablespoons Sugar Twin. Add 1 cup strawberries. Mix well to combine. Evenly spread mixture over bread in cake pan. Top with remaining slices of bread to form 4 sandwiches. In a large bowl, combine dry milk powder and 1 cup water. Add eggs and almond extract. Mix well to combine. Pour milk mixture evenly over sandwiches. Bake for 25 minutes or until golden brown. Meanwhile, in a medium saucepan, combine remaining 3 cups strawberries, remaining 6 tablespoons Sugar Twin, and remaining ¼ cup water. Cook over low heat, stirring occasionally, while toast is baking. For each serving, place 1 toasted sandwich on a plate, spoon a full ⅓ cup of warm strawberry sauce over top, and garnish with 1½ teaspoons almonds.

Each serving equals:

HE: 1½ Protein (½ limited) • 1 Bread • 1 Fruit • ½ Skim Milk • ¼ Fat • 19 Optional Calories

277 Calories • 5 gm Fat • 21 gm Protein • 37 gm Carbohydrate • 665 mg Sodium • 215 mg Calcium • 8 gm Fiber

DIABETIC: 1½ Meat • 1 Starch/Carbohydrate • 1 Fruit • ½ Skim Milk • ½ Fat

Peanut Butter Banana Muffins

When I say the words, "Peanut butter and banana," do you flash back to childhood and think of those messy but magnificent sandwiches of sliced bananas topped with crunchy peanut butter? I know I do. I still adore peanut butter and bananas, but now I savor that kid-pleasing flavor in a fresh and flavorful muffin!

○ Serves 12

> 1 cup + 2 tablespoons all-purpose flour
> ¾ cup (2¼ ounces) quick oats
> 1 tablespoon baking powder
> ¼ cup Brown Sugar Twin
> 1 cup (3 medium) mashed ripe bananas
>
> 1 cup skim milk
> ½ cup Peter Pan reduced-fat peanut butter
> 1 egg or equivalent in egg substitute
> 1 teaspoon vanilla extract

Preheat oven to 375 degrees. Spray the wells of a 12-hole muffin pan with butter-flavored cooking spray or line with paper liners. In a large bowl, combine flour, oats, baking powder, and Brown Sugar Twin. In a small bowl, combine bananas, skim milk, peanut butter, egg, and vanilla extract. Mix well using a wire whisk. Add banana mixture to flour mixture. Mix gently just to combine. Evenly spoon batter into prepared muffin wells. Bake for 16 to 18 minutes or until a toothpick inserted in center comes out clean. Place muffin pan on a wire rack and let set for 5 minutes. Remove muffins and continue cooling on wire rack.

Each serving equals:

HE: ¾ Bread • ¾ Protein • ⅔ Fat • ½ Fruit • 9 Optional Calories

152 Calories • 4 gm Fat • 6 gm Protein • 23 gm Carbohydrate • 188 mg Sodium • 100 mg Calcium • 2 gm Fiber

DIABETIC: 1 Starch • ½ Meat • ½ Fat • ½ Fruit

Cheesy Pizza Muffins

The kids are clamoring for pizza, but put down that phone! You can make pizza in a new, fun way with this quick and tangy recipe! The two kinds of cheese in these really double up the flavor.

◐ Serves 8

¼ cup finely chopped onion
¼ teaspoon dried minced garlic
1½ cups all-purpose flour
1 teaspoon Italian seasoning
2 teaspoons baking powder
¾ cup (3 ounces) shredded
    Kraft reduced-fat
    mozzarella cheese

¼ cup (1 ounce) sliced ripe
    olives
¾ cup tomato juice
1 egg, beaten, or equivalent in
    egg substitute
1 tablespoon olive oil
¼ cup (¾ ounce) grated Kraft
    fat-free Parmesan cheese

Preheat oven to 400 degrees. Spray 8 wells of a 12-hole muffin pan with olive oil–flavored cooking spray or line with paper liners. In a large bowl, combine onion, garlic, flour, Italian seasoning, and baking powder. Stir in mozzarella cheese and olives. In a small bowl, combine tomato juice, egg, and olive oil. Add liquid mixture to flour mixture. Mix just until moistened. Evenly spoon batter into prepared muffin wells. Sprinkle 1½ teaspoons Parmesan cheese evenly over top of each muffin. Bake for 20 to 25 minutes or until a toothpick inserted in center comes out clean. Place muffin pan on a wire rack and let set for 5 minutes. Remove muffins and continue cooling on wire rack.

HINT: Fill unused muffin wells with water. It protects the muffin pan and ensures even baking.

Each serving equals:

HE: 1 Bread • ¾ Protein • ½ Fat • ¼ Vegetable

---

161 Calories • 5 gm Fat • 7 gm Protein •
22 gm Carbohydrate • 353 mg Sodium •
157 mg Calcium • 1 gm Fiber

DIABETIC: 1 Starch • 1 Meat • ½ Fat

Maple-Apricot Bubble Loaf

If you've never nibbled a piece of "bubble" loaf, you're in for a real treat! These puffy rounds are sweet and fruity, and ready in just minutes. What a great dish to serve for a family reunion brunch!

○ Serves 6

1 (7.5-ounce) can Pillsbury refrigerated buttermilk biscuits
6 tablespoons apricot spreadable fruit
2 tablespoons Cary's Sugar Free Maple Syrup
3 tablespoons (¾ ounce) chopped pecans

Preheat oven to 375 degrees. Spray an 8-inch round cake pan with butter-flavored cooking spray. Separate biscuits and cut each into 4 pieces. Drop biscuit pieces into prepared cake pan. Lightly spray biscuit tops with butter-flavored cooking spray. In a medium bowl, combine spreadable fruit, maple syrup, and pecans. Spoon mixture evenly over biscuit pieces. Bake for 20 to 25 minutes or until golden brown. Place cake pan on a wire rack and let set for 5 minutes. Cut into 6 wedges. Serve warm.

Each serving equals:

HE: 1¼ Bread • 1 Fruit • ½ Fat • 3 Optional Calories

151 Calories • 3 gm Fat • 3 gm Protein •
28 gm Carbohydrate • 315 mg Sodium •
1 mg Calcium • 2 gm Fiber

DIABETIC: 1 Starch • 1 Fruit • ½ Fat

Easy Bruschetta

It's all the rage on restaurant menus, but now you can make this delectable dish at home! Topped with cheese, tomatoes, and Italian spices, these crusty squares have a spectacular appearance—and taste just as good!   ☺   Serves 8

1 (11-ounce) can Pillsbury Crusty French Loaf
1½ cups (6 ounces) shredded Kraft reduced-fat mozzarella cheese
1 tablespoon dried basil
1 teaspoon dried minced garlic
2 teaspoons dried parsley flakes
⅛ teaspoon black pepper
2 cups peeled and diced fresh tomatoes

Preheat oven to 375 degrees. Spray an 11-by-16-inch jelly roll pan with olive oil–flavored cooking spray. Unroll French loaf and pat dough into prepared pan and up sides of pan to form a rim. Lightly spray top with olive oil–flavored cooking spray. Bake for 5 minutes. Meanwhile, in a large bowl, combine mozzarella cheese, basil, garlic, parsley flakes, and black pepper. Add tomatoes. Toss gently to combine. Evenly sprinkle tomato mixture over partially baked crust. Continue baking for 8 to 10 minutes or until cheese melts. Cut into 8 pieces. Serve warm.

Each serving equals:

HE: 1 Protein • ⅔ Bread • ½ Vegetable

165 Calories • 5 gm Fat • 10 gm Protein •
20 gm Carbohydrate • 389 mg Sodium •
152 mg Calcium • 0 gm Fiber

DIABETIC: 1 Meat • 1 Starch • ½ Vegetable

Tomato Flat Bread

This is a great cocktail party appetizer, served up warm from your oven and oh-so-yummy! It looks so beautiful and challenging, people might think you hired a caterer, but tell them the truth—and accept all the cheers! ☻ Serves 8

½ cup finely chopped onion
½ cup Land O Lakes no-fat
    sour cream ☆
¼ cup Kraft fat-free
    mayonnaise
¾ cup (3 ounces) shredded
    Kraft reduced-fat
    Cheddar cheese

⅛ teaspoon black pepper
1 teaspoon Italian seasoning
1½ cups Bisquick Reduced Fat
    Baking Mix
⅓ cup skim milk
2½ cups peeled and chopped
    tomatoes
Dash paprika

Preheat oven to 400 degrees. Spray a rimmed 9-by-13-inch baking sheet with butter-flavored cooking spray. In a large skillet sprayed with butter-flavored cooking spray, sauté onion for 5 minutes. Remove from heat. Add 6 tablespoons sour cream, mayonnaise, Cheddar cheese, black pepper, and Italian seasoning. Mix well to combine. Set aside. In a large bowl, combine baking mix, skim milk, and remaining 2 tablespoons sour cream. Mix well to form a soft dough. Pat dough into prepared baking sheet. Evenly arrange tomatoes over dough. Spoon sour cream mixture evenly over tomatoes. Lightly sprinkle paprika over top. Bake for 20 to 25 minutes. Place baking sheet on a wire rack and let set for 5 minutes. Divide into 8 servings.

Each serving equals:

HE: 1 Bread • ¾ Vegetable • ½ Protein • ¼ Slider •
4 Optional Calories

152 Calories • 4 gm Fat • 6 gm Protein •
23 gm Carbohydrate • 457 mg Sodium •
134 mg Calcium • 1 gm Fiber

DIABETIC: 1 Starch • 1 Vegetable • ½ Meat

Dilly Cheese Biscuits

Even if you never fancied yourself much of a baker, this is the year you're going to do it! These biscuits are a great basic, perfect for serving to your family at a birthday supper, or for a dinner party of close friends. ☻ Serves 12

2¼ cups Bisquick Reduced Fat Baking Mix
1 tablespoon pourable Sugar Twin
1½ teaspoons dried dill weed
1 full cup (4½ ounces) shredded Kraft reduced-fat
    Cheddar cheese
1 cup skim milk
1 teaspoon prepared mustard
1 egg or equivalent in egg substitute

Preheat oven to 350 degrees. Spray the wells of a 12-hole muffin pan with butter-flavored cooking spray. In a large bowl, combine baking mix, Sugar Twin, dill weed, and Cheddar cheese. In a small bowl, combine skim milk, mustard, and egg. Add milk mixture to baking mix mixture. Mix well to combine. Evenly spoon batter into prepared muffin wells. Bake for 15 to 20 minutes or until a toothpick inserted in center comes out clean. Place muffin pan on a wire rack and let set for 5 minutes. Remove biscuits and continue cooling on wire rack.

Each serving equals:

HE: 1 Bread • ½ Protein • 13 Optional Calories

119 Calories • 3 gm Fat • 6 gm Protein •
17 gm Carbohydrate • 366 mg Sodium •
113 mg Calcium • 0 gm Fiber

DIABETIC: 1 Starch • ½ Meat

Cranberry Cornbread

There's just something so festive about a quick bread that features all those fruity bits of RED poking out from every slice! I'd serve this on Thanksgiving, but if bags of fresh cranberries are piled up at your local market, why not make a few loaves for holiday gifts?

Serves 8

> *1 cup (6 ounces) yellow cornmeal*
> *½ cup all-purpose flour*
> *¼ cup pourable Sugar Twin*
> *2 teaspoons baking powder*
> *½ teaspoon apple pie spice*
> *¼ teaspoon salt*
> *1½ cups chopped fresh cranberries*
> *¼ cup (1 ounce) chopped walnuts*
> *1¼ cups unsweetened applesauce*
> *1 egg or equivalent in egg substitute*

Preheat oven to 350 degrees. Spray an 8-by-8-inch baking dish with butter-flavored cooking spray. In a large bowl, combine cornmeal, flour, Sugar Twin, baking powder, apple pie spice, and salt. Stir in cranberries and walnuts. In a small bowl, combine applesauce and egg. Add applesauce mixture to cornmeal mixture. Mix gently just to combine. Spread mixture into prepared baking dish. Bake for 25 to 30 minutes or until a toothpick inserted in center comes out clean. Place baking dish on a wire rack and allow to cool. Cut into 8 pieces.

Each serving equals:

> HE: 1⅓ Bread • ½ Fruit • ¼ Protein • ¼ Fat • 3 Optional Calories
>
> _____
>
> 151 Calories • 3 gm Fat • 4 gm Protein •
> 27 gm Carbohydrate • 198 mg Sodium •
> 78 mg Calcium • 3 gm Fiber
>
> _____
>
> DIABETIC: 1½ Starch • ½ Fruit

Donut Balls

As a former donut gobbler, I was curious to see if I could figure out a healthy way to enjoy that irresistible donut taste. I hope you'll agree that these little "dough balls" come pretty close!

○ Serves 6 (2 each)

> 1 cup + 2 tablespoons Bisquick Reduced Fat Baking Mix
> ¼ cup + 2 tablespoons pourable Sugar Twin ☆
> 1 teaspoon ground cinnamon ☆
> 1 egg or equivalent in egg substitute
> ⅔ cup skim milk
> 1 teaspoon vanilla extract

Preheat oven to 375 degrees. Spray a 12-hole mini muffin pan with butter-flavored cooking spray. In a medium bowl, combine baking mix, ¼ cup Sugar Twin, and ½ teaspoon cinnamon. Add egg, skim milk, and vanilla extract. Mix well to combine. Drop by spoonfuls into prepared muffin pan. Bake for 14 to 16 minutes. Place muffin pan on a wire rack and cool for 10 minutes. Remove balls from pan. In a Ziploc plastic bag, combine remaining 2 tablespoons Sugar Twin and remaining ½ teaspoon cinnamon. Place donuts in bag, 2 or 3 at a time, and shake to coat.

Each serving equals:

HE: 1 Bread • ¼ Slider • 6 Optional Calories

102 Calories • 2 gm Fat • 4 gm Protein •
17 gm Carbohydrate • 286 mg Sodium •
59 mg Calcium • 0 gm Fiber

DIABETIC: 1 Starch /Carbohydrate

Golden Treasures

Are these candies or cookies? Hmm . . . Wait—does it really matter as long as they taste terrific? 🙂 Serves 6 (3 each)

2 tablespoons Peter Pan reduced-fat chunky peanut butter
⅔ cup Carnation Nonfat Dry Milk Powder
2 tablespoons pourable Sugar Twin
⅓ cup Cary's Sugar Free Maple Syrup
1 teaspoon vanilla extract
1½ cups (4½ ounces) quick oats

Arrange wax paper on 2 baking sheets. In a large bowl, combine peanut butter, dry milk powder, Sugar Twin, maple syrup, and vanilla extract. Stir in oats. Drop mixture by tablespoonful onto prepared baking sheets to form 18 balls. Refrigerate for at least 30 minutes. Cover and refrigerate leftovers.

Each serving equals:

HE: 1 Bread • ⅓ Skim Milk • ⅓ Protein • ⅓ Fat • 11 Optional Calories

---

143 Calories • 3 gm Fat • 7 gm Protein • 22 gm Carbohydrate • 97 mg Sodium • 102 mg Calcium • 2 gm Fiber

---

DIABETIC: 1 Starch/Carbohydrate • 1 Fat

Chocolate Cereal Mounds

When the kids come home after school and want a sweet treat, here's a way to satisfy their appetites but know you've given them something good for them, too! ☻ Serves 8 (4 each)

> 1 (4-serving) package JELL-O sugar-free chocolate cook-and-serve
>   pudding mix
> ½ cup water
> ¼ cup Peter Pan reduced-fat peanut butter
> ¾ cup (1½ ounces) miniature marshmallows
> 1 tablespoon vanilla extract
> 1½ cups (4½ ounces) uncooked quick oats
> ¼ cup (1 ounce) chopped dry roasted peanuts

Arrange wax paper on 2 baking sheets. In a medium saucepan, combine dry pudding mix and water. Stir in peanut butter. Cook over medium heat until mixture thickens and starts to boil, stirring constantly. Stir in marshmallows and vanilla extract. Continue cooking until mixture is smooth, stirring constantly. Remove from heat. Add oats and peanuts. Mix well to combine. Drop mixture by tablespoonful onto prepared baking sheets to form 32 mounds. Refrigerate for at least 30 minutes. Cover and refrigerate leftovers.

Each serving equals:

HE: ¾ Bread • ¾ Fat • ⅔ Protein • ¼ Slider •
2 Optional Calories

157 Calories • 5 gm Fat • 6 gm Protein •
22 gm Carbohydrate • 95 mg Sodium •
10 mg Calcium • 2 gm Fiber

DIABETIC: 1 Starch • 1 Fat • 1 Meat

Strawberry Banana Float

This was so delicious, I had to keep testing it—just to be sure! Why, I think I tested this recipe every day for a week! Now, *you* don't have to, but you might be persuaded to enjoy it VERY often.

☻ Serves 4

> *2 cups Wells' Blue Bunny strawberry sugar- and fat-free ice cream*
>   *or any sugar- and fat-free ice cream ☆*
> *1½ cups sliced fresh strawberries*
> *⅓ cup (1 medium) mashed ripe banana*
> *1⅓ cups skim milk ☆*
> *¼ cup unsweetened orange juice*
> *¼ cup Cool Whip Lite*

In a blender container, combine 1½ cups ice cream, strawberries, banana, and ⅓ cup skim milk. Cover and process on BLEND for 20 seconds. Add remaining 1 cup skim milk and orange juice. Re-cover and continue processing on BLEND until mixture is smooth. Pour mixture evenly into 4 glasses. Top each glass with 2 tablespoons ice cream and 1 tablespoon Cool Whip Lite.

Each serving equals:

> HE: 1 Fruit • ⅓ Skim Milk • ¾ Slider •
> 15 Optional Calories
> _____
> 161 Calories • 1 gm Fat • 8 gm Protein •
> 30 gm Carbohydrate • 114 mg Sodium •
> 270 mg Calcium • 1 gm Fiber
> _____
> DIABETIC: 1 Fruit • 1 Starch/Carbohydrate

Lemon Berry Fizz

It's sweet! It's tart! It's fizzy and fantastic! It's the perfect beverage to serve at your next backyard barbecue! How can anything this delicious be so low-calorie and easy?   ◐   Serves 8 (1 cup)

2 cups cold water
1 tub Crystal Light sugar-free lemonade mix
4 cups Ocean Spray reduced-calorie cranberry juice cocktail
2 cups diet ginger ale

In a large container, combine water and dry lemonade mix. Add cranberry juice cocktail and ginger ale. Mix well to combine. Serve over ice.

Each serving equals:

HE: ½ Fruit

28 Calories • 0 gm Fat • 0 gm Protein •
7 gm Carbohydrate • 27 mg Sodium •
2 mg Calcium • 0 gm Fiber

DIABETIC: ½ Fruit

Sangria Spritzer

Every time I start to experiment with new non-alcoholic beverage recipes, it seems that everyone gathers around to sip and sample them! My testers agreed that this sparkling fruit punch was spectacular! ☻ Serves 4 (1 full cup)

> 1 cup unsweetened grape juice
> ½ cup unsweetened orange juice
> 3 tablespoons lemon juice
> 3 tablespoons lime juice
> 2¼ cups diet ginger ale

In a pitcher, combine grape juice, orange juice, lemon juice, and lime juice. Refrigerate for at least 1 hour. Just before serving, stir in diet ginger ale. Serve over ice.

HINT: Attractive garnished with an orange slice.

Each serving equals:

HE: 1 Fruit

---

64 Calories • 0 gm Fat • 1 gm Protein •
15 gm Carbohydrate • 23 mg Sodium •
13 mg Calcium • 0 gm Fiber

DIABETIC: 1 Fruit

Acapulco Sunshine

Instead of a glass of OJ tomorrow morning, why not start your day with a blast of flavor from south of the border? This sunny, citrusy beverage will energize you and tickle your tastebuds.

🌀 Serves 4 (1 scant cup)

> *1 cup unsweetened orange juice*
> *1 cup (one 8-ounce can) crushed pineapple, packed in fruit juice, undrained*
> *1¼ cups Diet Mountain Dew*
> *1 cup crushed ice*
> *4 maraschino cherries*

In a blender container, combine orange juice, undrained pineapple, and Diet Mountain Dew. Cover and process on BLEND for 30 seconds. Add ice. Re-cover and continue processing on BLEND for 30 seconds or until mixture is smooth. Pour into glasses. Garnish each glass rim with a maraschino cherry.

Each serving equals:

HE: 1 Fruit • 10 Optional Calories

72 Calories • 0 gm Fat • 0 gm Protein •
18 gm Carbohydrate • 8 mg Sodium •
14 mg Calcium • 0 gm Fiber

DIABETIC: 1 Fruit

Applesauce Milk Shake

This is a category of recipe I call "Why Not?" Everyone loves creamy milkshakes; everyone adores sweet and spicy applesauce. Why not stir them up together and launch a beautiful friendship!

○ Serves 4 (¾ cup)

> 1 cup skim milk
> 1 cup Wells' Blue Bunny sugar- and fat-free vanilla ice cream or
>   any sugar- and fat-free ice cream
> 1 cup unsweetened applesauce
> ½ teaspoon apple pie spice

In a blender container, combine skim milk, ice cream, applesauce, and apple pie spice. Cover and process on BLEND for 20 to 30 seconds or until smooth. Serve at once.

Each serving equals:

HE: ½ Fruit • ¼ Skim Milk • ¼ Slider •
10 Optional Calories

---

92 Calories • 0 gm Fat • 4 gm Protein •
19 gm Carbohydrate • 58 mg Sodium •
137 mg Calcium • 1 gm Fiber

DIABETIC: ½ Fruit •
½ Starch/Carbohydrate or 1 Starch/Carbohydrate

Cran-Orange Refresher

This fruit shake turns a glorious color when the blender goes to work, but it's the taste that will win you over! Now, don't delay—serve it right away!   ☻   Serves 4 (¾ cup)

> 1½ cups Ocean Spray reduced-calorie cranberry juice cocktail
> ¾ cup unsweetened orange juice
> 2 cups Wells' Blue Bunny sugar- and fat-free vanilla ice cream or any sugar- and fat-free ice cream

In a blender container, combine cranberry juice cocktail and orange juice. Cover and process on BLEND for 5 seconds. Add ice cream. Re-cover and continue processing on BLEND for 10 to 15 seconds or until mixture is smooth. Serve at once.

Each serving equals:

HE: ¾ Fruit • ½ Slider • 10 Optional Calories

124 Calories • 0 gm Fat • 4 gm Protein •
27 gm Carbohydrate • 64 mg Sodium •
124 mg Calcium • 1 gm Fiber

DIABETIC: 1 Fruit • 1 Starch/Carbohydrate

Menus to Inspire a Return to Good Health

Enjoying the Wonder of Winter Brunch
Cranberry Cornbread
Apple Scrapple
Asparagus Brunch Bake
Secret Skillet Potatoes
Carrot Cake Cookies

Savoring the Splendor of Spring Supper
Orange Spinach Salad
Tulip Time Rhubarb Salad
Sunshine State Simmered Steaks
Dixie Chocolate Mayonnaise Cake
Lemon Berry Fizz

"Better Than Ever" Summer Birthday Party
Strawberry Lemon Gelatin Salad
Creamy Cauliflower and Broccoli Salad
Diane's Angel Hair Pasta and Chicken
White Chocolate Raspberry Cheesecake
Cran-Orange Refresher

"Together Forever" Anniversary Dinner
Baby Quiche Appetizers
Easy Vegetables Alfredo
Italian Pepper Steak
Black Tie Chocolate Cheesecake
Sangria Spritzer

Finding the Glory in Fall Leaf-Raking Potluck
Lone Star Corn Chili
Oktoberfest Red Cabbage Salad
Eggplant Parmesan
Enchilada Casserole
Easy Pumpkin Raisin Pie

Gathering Family and Friends for a Holiday Buffet
Grandma's Soup Pot
Broccoli Harvest Salad
Hawaiian Meatloaf
Calico Potato and Ham Bake
Holiday Orange Cheesecake with Cranberry Glaze

Making Healthy Exchanges Work for You

You're ready now to begin a wonderful journey to better health. In the preceding pages, you've discovered the remarkable variety of good food available to you when you begin eating the *Healthy Exchanges Way*. You've stocked your pantry and learned many of my food preparation "secrets" that will point you on the way to delicious success.

But before I let you go, I'd like to share a few tips that I've learned while traveling toward healthier eating habits. It took me a long time to learn how to eat *smarter*. In fact, I'm still working on it. But I am getting better. For years, I could *inhale* a five-course meal in five minutes flat—and still make room for a second helping of dessert!

Now I follow certain signposts on the road that help me stay on the right path. I hope these ideas will help point you in the right direction as well.

1. **Eat slowly** so your brain has time to catch up with your tummy. Cut and chew each bite slowly. Try putting your fork down between bites. Stop eating as soon as you feel full. Crumple your napkin and throw it on top of your plate so you don't continue to eat when you are no longer hungry.

2. **Smaller plates** may help you feel more satisfied by your food portions *and* limit the amount you can put on the plate.

3. **Watch portion size.** If you are *truly* hungry, you can always add more food to your plate once you've finished your initial serving. But remember to count the additional food accordingly.

4. **Always eat at your dining-room or kitchen table.** You deserve better than nibbling from an open refrigerator or over the sink. Make an attractive place setting, even if you're eating alone. Feed your eyes as well as your stomach. By always eating at a table, you will become much more aware of your true food intake. For some reason, many of us conveniently "forget" the food we swallow while standing over the stove or munching in the car or on the run.

5. **Avoid doing anything else while you are eating.** If you read the paper or watch television while you eat, it's easy to consume too much food without realizing it, because you are concentrating on something else besides what you're eating. Then, when you look down at your plate and see that it's empty, you wonder where all the food went and why you still feel hungry.

Day by day, as you travel the path to good health, it will become easier to make the right choices, to eat *smarter*. But don't ever fool yourself into thinking that you'll be able to put your eating habits on cruise control and forget about them. Making a commitment to eat good healthy food and sticking to it takes some effort. But with all the good-tasting recipes in this Healthy Exchanges cookbook, just think how well you're going to eat—and enjoy it—from now on!

Healthy Lean Bon Appétit!

Index

C

I want to hear from you . . .

Besides my family, the love of my life is creating "common folk" healthy recipes and solving everyday cooking questions in the *Healthy Exchanges Way*. Everyone who uses my recipes is considered part of the Healthy Exchanges Family, so please write to me if you have any questions, comments, or suggestions. I will do my best to answer. With your support, I'll continue to stir up even more recipes and cooking tips for the Family in the years to come.

> Write to: JoAnna M. Lund
> c/o Healthy Exchanges, Inc.
> P.O. Box 124
> DeWitt, IA 52742

If you prefer, you can fax me at 1-319-659-2126 or contact me via e-mail by writing to HealthyJo@aol.com. Or visit my Healthy Exchanges Internet web site at: http://www.healthyexchanges.com.

About the Author

JOANNA M. LUND, a graduate of the University of Western Illinois, worked as a commercial insurance underwriter for eighteen years before starting her own business, Healthy Exchanges, Inc., which publishes cookbooks, a monthly newsletter, motivational booklets, and inspirational audiotapes. Her first book, *Healthy Exchanges Cookbook,* has more than 500,000 copies in print. A popular speaker with hospitals, support groups for heart patients and diabetics, and service and volunteer organizations, she appears regularly on QVC and on regional television and radio shows, and has been featured in newspapers and magazines across the country. She has also hosted a 26-episode series for public television, *Help Yourself with JoAnna Lund.*

The recipient of numerous business awards, JoAnna was an Iowa delegate to the national White House Conference on Small Business. She is a member of the International Association of Culinary Professionals, the Society for Nutritional Education, and other professional publishing and marketing associations. She lives with her husband, Clifford, in DeWitt, Iowa.

CATHERINE A. MUHA, R.N, M.S.N., is a Clinical Specialist in Oncology at the National Cancer Institute, which is part of the National Institutes of Health in Bethesda, Maryland. She works in health communications research for the Cancer Information Service, a national referral service for cancer patients, based at the National Cancer Institute.

The Cancer Information Service at the National Cancer Institute can be reached at 1-800-4-CANCER.

Now That You've Seen
The Cancer Recovery Healthy Exchanges Cookbook, Why Not Order The Healthy Exchanges Food Newsletter?

If you enjoyed the recipes in this cookbook and would like to cook up even more of these "common folk" healthy dishes, you may want to subscribe to *The Healthy Exchanges Food Newsletter*.

This monthly 12-page newsletter contains 30-plus new recipes *every month,* in such columns as:

- Reader Exchange
- Reader Requests
- Recipe Makeover
- Micro Corner
- Dinner for Two

- Crock-Pot Luck
- Meatless Main Dishes
- Rise & Shine
- Our Small World

- Brown Bagging It
- Snack Attack
- Side Dishes
- Main Dishes
- Desserts

In addition to all the recipes, other regular features include:

- The Editor's Motivational Corner
- Dining Out Question & Answer
- Cooking Question & Answer
- New Product Alert
- Success Profiles of Winners in the Losing Game
- Exercise Advice from a Cardiac Rehab Specialist
- Nutrition Advice from a Registered Dietitian
- Positive Thought for the Month

Just as in this cookbook, all *Healthy Exchanges Food Newsletter* recipes are calculated in three distinct ways: 1) Weight Loss Choices, 2) Calories with Fat and Fiber Grams, and 3) Diabetic Exchanges.

The cost for a one-year (12-issue) subscription is $22.50. To order, simply complete the form and mail to us *or* call our toll-free number and pay with your VISA or MasterCard.

_____ Yes, I want to subscribe to *The Healthy Exchanges Food Newsletter*

$22.50 Yearly Subscription Cost . . . . $_____

Foreign orders please add $6.00 for money exchange and extra postage . . . . $_____

_____ I'm not sure, so please send me a sample copy at $2.50 . . . . $_____

Please make check payable to HEALTHY EXCHANGES or pay by VISA / MasterCard

CARD NUMBER: _____ EXPIRATION DATE: _____

SIGNATURE: _____
   Signature required for all credit card orders.

Or Order Toll-Free, using your credit card, at 1-800-766-8961

NAME: _____

ADDRESS: _____

CITY: _____ STATE: _____ ZIP: _____

TELEPHONE: (_____) _____

If additional orders for the newsletter are to be sent to an address other than the one listed above, please use a separate sheet and attach to this form.

MAIL TO: **HEALTHY EXCHANGES**
   P.O. BOX 124
   DeWitt, IA 52742-0124

   1-800-766-8961 for customer orders
   1-319-659-8234 for customer service

Thank you for your order, and for choosing to become a part of the Healthy Exchanges Family!